Liver Cancer - Simple Approach

With Orthodox and Alternative Treatment

Preface

I have written this book so that the patients suffering from Liver cancer can understand the disease in detail and choose a suitable treatment for them. This book provides simple approach about the clinical symptoms, complications, diagnosis, staging and treatments. In the last 15 years there has been considerable research and progress in the field of clinical studies, etiology, pathology, diagnosis and treatment of Liver cancer.

In this book, I have written in detail about Orthodox and Alternative Treatment (Budwig Protocol, which is the best alternative treatment and gives authentic success). Patient can carefully select the right treatment for him. This book has up to date information.

Dr. O.P.Verma

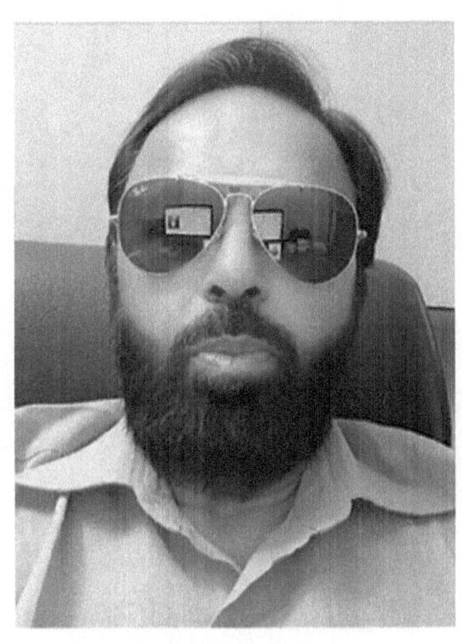

Written by
Dr. O.P.Verma
M.B.B.S., M.R.S.H. (London)
Budwig Wellness
7-B-43, Mahaveer Nagar III, Kota (Raj.)
https://gobudwig.com
+919460816360

Table of Content

Facts about Liver

Human liver is a very vital organ. It is so important that if it stops functioning even for a single day, a person will simply die. Unfortunately, it is one of the least thought about organs. So, it is time that we change our view and start giving it the much deserved attention. Here are some interesting facts about human liver.

1. The size of the liver increases with age, from an average span of 5 cm at the age of five years, to 15 cm in adulthood. The normal liver weighs 1.4 to 1.5 kg in men and 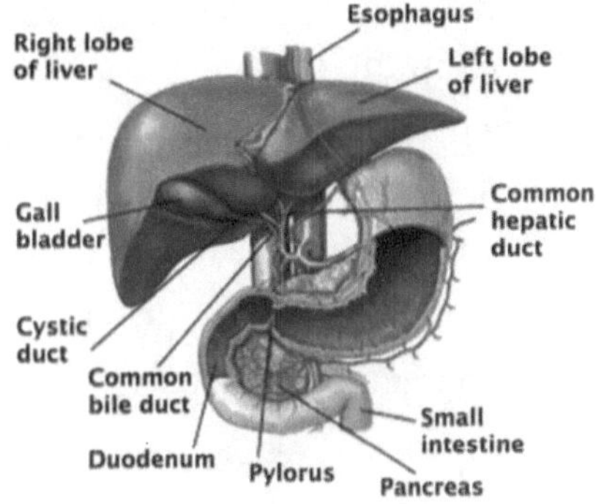

1.2 to 1.4 kg in women and is reddish-brown in color. The liver has two main lobes – the right lobe and the left lobe. The right lobe is bigger than the left lobe and has two small lobes on visceral surface of right lobe, caudate lobe and quadrate lobe.

2. 'Hepar' is the Greek term for liver. It is because of this Greek name that most liver related medical terms actually start with 'hepatic or hepato'.

3. Liver protects our body from harmful substances or toxin that we put in our body either deliberately or unintentionally through food we eat or drink.

4. The liver also protects our body from the toxins by cleaning the blood from chemicals that spontaneously enter within our body because of day to day activities.

5. The chemicals removed from the blood are sent into our intestines in form of bile. These chemicals are then removed in form of feces or stool. These chemicals may also be sent into the kidneys where they are filtered out from the body in form of urine.

6. Liver is responsible for producing bile. Bile is very important because it helps in digesting food. Of course, without bile the body would simply fail to remove toxins from the body.

7. The bile produced by the liver is also important because it helps to breakdown fats into smaller particles so that the pancreatic lipase can digest fat better.

8. Bile produced by liver is also responsible for the characteristic brown color of the stool.

9. Our body produces a chemical known as bilirubin. This is a toxic substance and if it goes unfiltered into the kidneys, it can damage them. The liver actually conjugates bilirubin and excrete in bile. Intestinal bacteria convert bilirubin to urobilinogen. Small amount of urobilinogen enters in kidney and excreted in urine as urobilin. This is what gives the characteristic yellow color to our urine.

10. Humans are not the only living beings to have a liver, rather any living creature with a spinal column or a backbone has a liver. In short every vertebrate in this world has a liver.

11. The Greeks considered the liver to be the home of all human emotions. According to Greeks, the liver was the organ which was closest to divine presence.

12. Yet, another interesting fact about liver is that it never uses sugar for energy. It only stores sugar. In reality, liver is the storehouse of any excess sugar that we consume. It stores this sugar in form of a compound known as glycogen. Between meals when our body needs sugar, the liver breaks down the glycogen to form glucose. This glucose is then used by the remaining body as an energy source.

13. Almost all medicines that we consume are processed by the liver. Because our body is not capable of using the medicines as is, the liver breaks them down in a form that the body can use.

14. The liver is responsible for producing enzymes and chemicals that helps the blood to clot in the event of bleeding due to a cut.

15. Liver is also responsible for making cholesterol. While high levels of low density lipoprotein or (bad cholesterol) is actually bad, cholesterol is also required for building cells as well as hormones. Hormones are necessary for normal functioning of the body because they can be rightly termed as the messengers in our body. Absence of hormones will lead to abnormal body functioning because they will fail to communicate properly.

16. Liver is responsible for performing over 500 different vital functions of the body.

17. At any given point in time, liver contains 10% of the total blood in the body. It filters around 1.4 liters of blood every single minute.

18. The Greeks used to practice what we today call as hepatoscopy. It is a practice where the Greeks used to sacrifice goats and oxen and examined their livers to

determine whether they will earn victory in a battle or war.

19. Human liver is actually an iron warehouse. It also contains extra minerals and vitamins which allows a person to perform throughout the day.

20. Our body that is up and running is because of the blood. If blood wasn't there right from the beginning, we would not even exist. This blood was actually made by liver even before our birth.

21. Yes, we did say that artificial liver replacement is not possible but liver transplant is possible. One very interesting fact about liver is that it can sustain and survive heavy damage. It can grow back.

22. Liver transplant usually involves cutting out a certain part of the liver from the donor and giving it to the receiver. The part of the liver that is cut out from the donor can actually grow back!

23. The first ever liver transplant in human history was carried out by Dr. Thomas E. Starzl in year 1963 at University of Colorado Medical School. The transplant was not successful because of the lack of effective immunosuppressive drugs. He made another attempt in 1967 and the transplant was successful.

Anatomy of Liver

The liver is a peritoneal organ positioned in the right upper part (quadrant) of the abdomen. It is the largest visceral structure in the abdominal cavity and the largest gland in the human body, weighing in at around 3 pounds.

An accessory digestion gland, the liver performs a wide range of functions; including synthesis of bile, glycogen storage and clotting factor production.

The posterior aspect of the diaphragmatic surface is not covered by visceral peritoneum, and is in direct contact with the diaphragm itself (known as the 'bare area' of the liver).

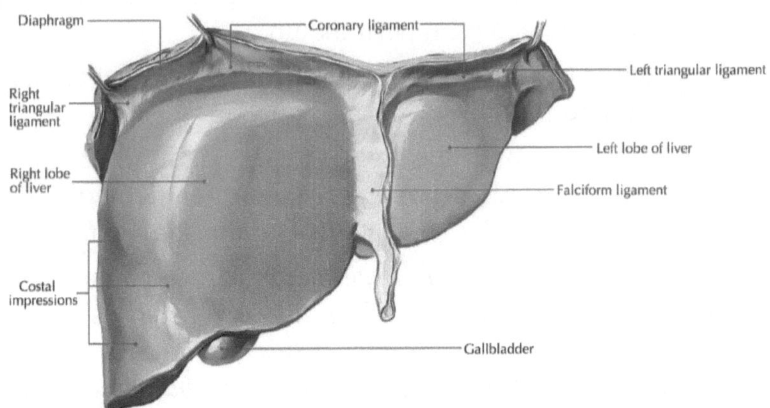

Anatomical Position

The liver is predominantly located in the right hypochondrium and epigastric areas, and extends into the left hypochondrium.

When discussing the anatomical position of the liver, it is useful to consider its external surfaces, associated ligaments, and the anatomical spaces (recesses) that surround it.

Liver Surfaces

The external surfaces of the liver are described by their location and adjacent structures. There are two liver surfaces – the diaphragmatic (which is in contact with diaphragm, dome-shaped, structure that separates the chest and abdomen) and visceral:

Diaphragmatic surface – the anterosuperior surface of the liver.

It is smooth and convex, fitting snugly beneath the curvature of the diaphragm.

Visceral surface – the posteroinferior surface of the liver.

With the exception of the fossa of the gallbladder and porta hepatis, it is covered with peritoneum.

It is moulded by the shape of the surrounding organs, making it irregular and flat.

It lies in contact with the right kidney, right adrenal gland, right colic flexure, transverse colon, first part of the duodenum, gallbladder, esophagus and the stomach.

It should be noted that the peritoneum is a serous membrane forming the lining of the abdominal cavity and covers most of the intra-abdominal organs. It has two layers. The outer layer, the parietal peritoneum, lines the abdominal and the pelvic walls and the inner layer, the visceral peritoneum, is wrapped around the visceral organs.

Ligaments of the Liver

There are various ligaments that attach the liver to the surrounding structures. These are formed by a double layer of peritoneum.

Falciform ligament – This sickle-shaped ligament attaches the anterior surface of the liver to the anterior abdominal wall and forms a natural anatomical division between the left and right lobs of the liver. The free edge of this ligament contains the ligamentum teres, a remnant of the umbilical vein.

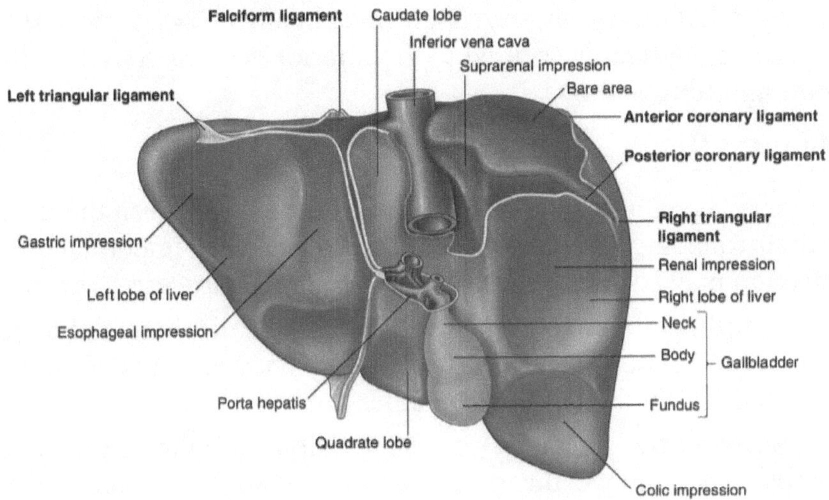

Coronary ligament (anterior and posterior folds) – attaches the superior surface of the liver to the inferior surface of the diaphragm and demarcates the bare area of the liver The anterior and posterior folds unite to form the triangular ligaments on the right and left lobes of the liver.

Triangular ligaments (left and right):

The left triangular ligament is formed by the union of the anterior and posterior layers of the coronary ligament at the apex of the liver and attaches the left lobe of the liver to the diaphragm.

The right triangular ligament is formed in a similar fashion adjacent to the bare area and attaches the right lobe of the liver to the diaphragm.

Lesser omentum – Attaches the liver to the lesser curvature of the stomach and first part of the duodenum. It consists of the hepatoduodenal ligament (extends from the duodenum to the liver) and the hepatogastric ligament (extends from the stomach to the liver). The hepatoduodenal ligament surrounds the portal triad.

In addition to these supporting ligaments, the posterior surface of the liver is secured to the inferior vena cava by hepatic veins and fibrous tissue.

Hepatic Recesses

The hepatic recesses are anatomical spaces between the liver and surrounding structures. They are of clinical importance as infection may collect in these areas, forming an abscess.

Subphrenic spaces – located between the diaphragm and the anterior and superior aspects of the liver. They are divided into a right and left by the falciform ligament.

Subhepatic space – a subdivision of the supracolic compartment (above the transverse mesocolon), this peritoneal space is located between the inferior surface of the liver and the transverse colon.

Morison's pouch – a potential space between the visceral surface of the liver and the right kidney. This is the deepest part of the peritoneal cavity when someone is lying flat, therefore pathological abdominal fluid such as blood or ascites is most likely to collect in this region in a bedridden patient.

Anatomical Structure

The structure of the liver can be considered both macroscopically and microscopically.

Macroscopic

The liver is covered by a fibrous layer, known as Glisson's capsule.

It is divided into a right lobe and left lobe by the attachment of the falciform ligament. There are two further 'accessory' lobes that arise from the right lobe, and are located on the visceral surface of liver:

Caudate lobe – located on the upper aspect of the visceral surface. It lies between the inferior vena cava and a fossa produced by the ligamentum venosum (a remnant of the fetal ductus venosus).

Quadrate lobe – located on the lower aspect of the visceral surface. It lies between the gallbladder and a fossa produced by the ligamentum teres (a remnant of the fetal umbilical vein).

Separating the caudate and quadrate lobes is a deep, transverse fissure – known as the porta hepatis. It transmits all the vessels, nerves and ducts entering or leaving the liver with the exception of the hepatic veins.

Microscopic structure of Liver

To understand the function of the liver it is necessary to understand the blood supply to the liver. It is supplied by the hepatic artery in the typical manner but it is the only digestive organ drained by the inferior vena cava. Other digestive organs such as the small intestine, parts of the large intestine, stomach and pancreas are drained by the hepatic portal system which takes the blood directly to the liver. Thus, the liver receives oxygen poor, nutrient rich blood from the hepatic portal system and oxygen rich blood from the hepatic artery.

The liver consists of the following major histological components:

Stroma - which is a continuation of the surrounding capsule of Glisson. It consists of connective tissue and contains the vessels. The capsule is also covered by a layer of mesothelium, arising from the peritoneum covering the liver. The connective tissue of the stroma is type III collagen (reticulin), which forms a meshwork that provides integrity for the hepatocytes and sinusoids.

Parenchyma - which is mainly represented by hepatocytes

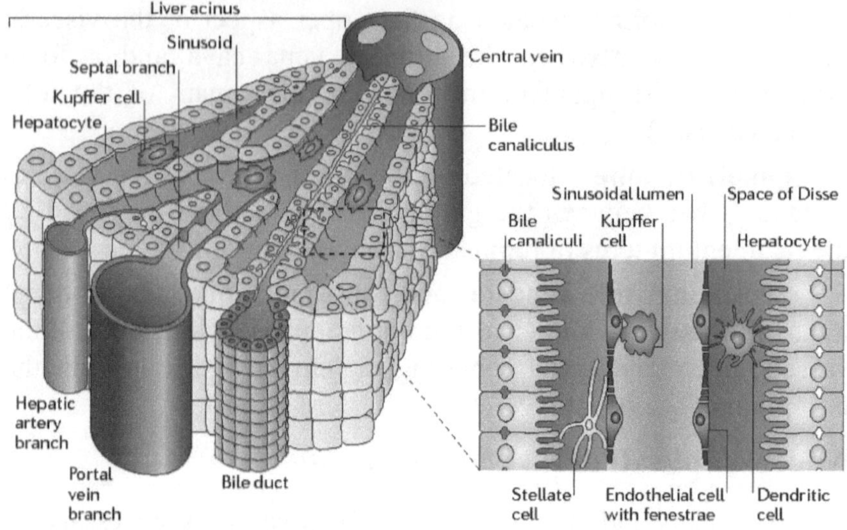

Hepatocytes

The internal structure of the liver is made of around 100,000 small hexagonal functional units known as lobules. Hepatocytes are one of the primary functional cells of the liver. These large and polyhedral (six surfaces) cells make up 80% of the total cells of the liver. They can contain between two and four nuclei, which are large and spherical, occupying the centre of the cells. Each nucleus has at least two nucleoli. The typical lifespan of a hepatocyte is five months. They are located in flat irregular plates that are arranged radially like the spokes of a wheel around a branch of the hepatic vein, called the central vein or central venule since it really has the structure of a venule. The adjacent hepatocytes leave a very small space between them known as bile canaliculi which are almost 1.0-2.0 μm in diameter. The cell membranes near these canaliculi are joined by tight junctions.

10

These rows are one cell wide and are surrounded by sinusoidal capillaries or sinusoids. This arrangement ensures that each hepatocyte is in very close contact with blood flowing through the sinusoids, i.e. bathed in blood.

The endothelial cells lining sinusoids are fenestrated and in most species lack a basal lamina. Gaps are also present between the endothelial cells. Taken together these two properties make the sinusoids extremely leaky and allow for the extremely close contact between the blood and the surface of hepatocytes. Many materials in the blood, except for whole blood cells, can pass between the spaces in the sinusoidal lining.

Although sinudoidal endothelial cells lie very close to hepatocytes, they do not actually make contact. A narrow space is present between the surface of the hepatocyte and the surface of the endothelial cell. This is called the **space of Disse**; it is filled with numerous microvilli from the hepatocytes. As in other areas of the body, these microvilli serve to increase the surface area of the cell membrane that comes in contact with the blood facilitating exchange of molecules between hepatocytes and the blood.

In addition, sinusoids contain a specific cell type called **Kupffer cell**, containing ovoid nuclei. These monocyte derivatives of the mononuclear phagocytic system are part of the sinusoid lining from which they extend processes into the lumen.

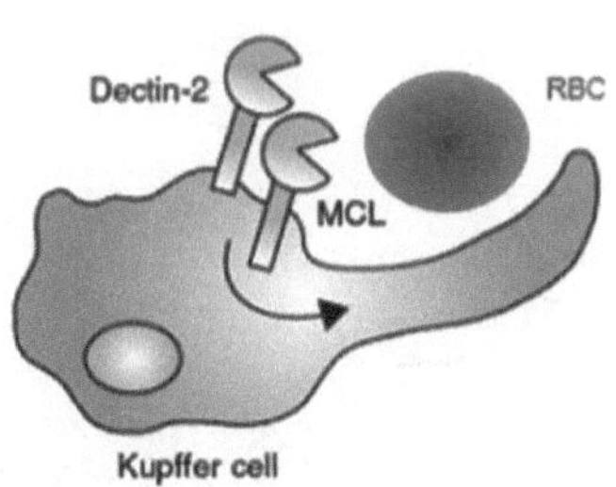

Therefore, Kupffer cells continuously sample the blood travelling through the sinusoids, phagocytosing antigens, microorganisms, and damaged red blood cells.

The cytoplasm is acidophilic in routine H&E staining, dotted with basophilic regions represented by rough endoplasmic reticulum (rER) and ribosomes. In addition, hepatocytes contain the following organelles:

- Smooth endoplasmic reticulum (sER), which is essential in toxin degradation and conjugation, as well as cholesterol synthesis.

- Mitochondria (up to 1000/cell)

- Golgi network, which is composed of approximately 50 small Golgi units. They contain granules with very low density lipoprotein and bile precursors.

- Peroxisomes, which contain oxidases and catalases. These enzymes are responsible for detoxification reactions taking place in the liver, for example, that of alcohol.

- Glycogen deposits, which are lost in during H&E preparations, leaving irregular stained areas.

- Lipid droplets

- Lysosomes, which are responsible for iron storage under the form of ferritin.

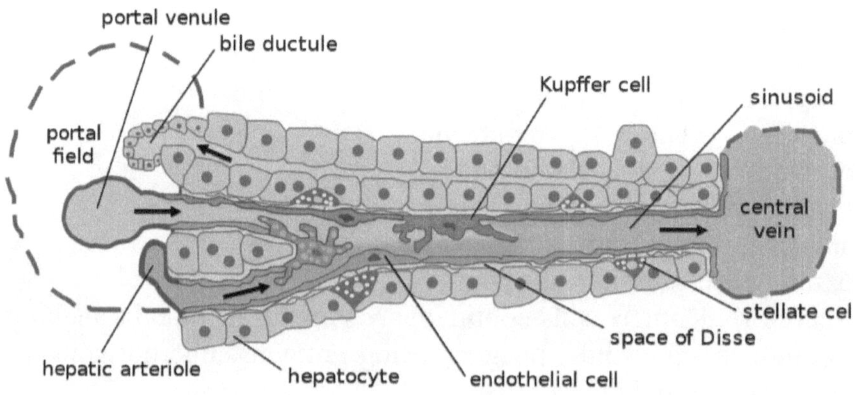

The perisinusoidal space contains a specific type of cell called **Ito, or hepatic stellate cells.** Their role is the storage of hepatic vitamin A inside lipid droplets, which is subsequently released as retinol. However, Ito cells are also responsible for hepatic fibrosis, since they are the ones secreting large amounts of collagen during liver injury.

Hepatic Lobules

In histological terms, the liver consists of a large number of microscopic functional units that work in unison to ensure the overall, proper activity of the entire organ. View the enclosed pictures to appreciate and understand the microscopic architecture of liver lobules. There are three possible ways of describing one such unit, as given below:

Classic Hepatic lobule

The classic lobule is the traditional description and the one that you have most likely heard of the most. It consists of hexagonal plates of hepatocytes stacked on top of each other. Within each plate, the hepatocytes radiate outwards from a central vein. As they extend towards the periphery, the hepatocytes are arranged into strips, similar to the spokes of a cartwheel. Hepatic sinusoids travel between the strips of hepatocytes, draining into the central vein.

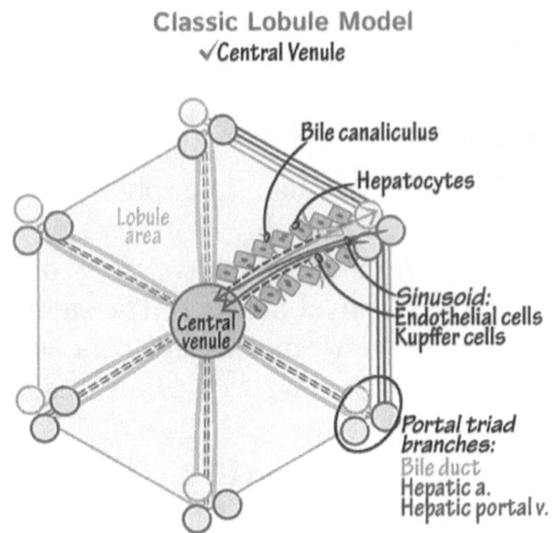

One portal canal is located at each corner of the hexagonal classic lobule, making a total of six for each lobule. These portal canals are composed of the portal triads, which are surrounded by loose stromal connective tissue. A periportal space (space of Mall), where lymph is produced, is sandwiched between the connective tissue of the portal canals and the hepatocytes.

While connective tissue is present around the portal canals, the interlobular quantity is very small in humans. This can make routine histological visualizations of the classic lobule difficult.

Portal lobule

While the classic lobule view focuses on the blood supply and hepatic mass arrangement, the portal lobule view underlines the exocrine function of the liver i.e. bile secretion. In this case, each functional unit is a triangle, having a central axis through a portal canal and the imaginary vertices through the three different but closest portal canals surrounding it. The area covered by the triangle represents the hepatic regions that secrete bile into the same bile duct. The flow of bile is from periphery to the center into the bile ductile.

Liver acinus

The focus of this description is the oxygen saturation, metabolism and pathology of hepatocytes, providing a more accurate description of the physiology of the liver. A liver acinus functional unit is oval in shape. The short axis is represented by a shared border between two adjacent lobules together with the portal canals. The long axis is an imaginary line between two adjacent central veins.

Each liver acinus can be divided into three zones:

Zone 1 - It is the one closest to the short axis, hence to the portal canals and supply of arterial blood. The hepatocytes in zone 1 receive the highest amount of oxygen.

Zone 2 - It is the one located between zones 1 and 3.

Zone 3 - It is the one furthest from the short axis but closest to the central vein, hence the hepatocytes receive the least amount of oxygen.

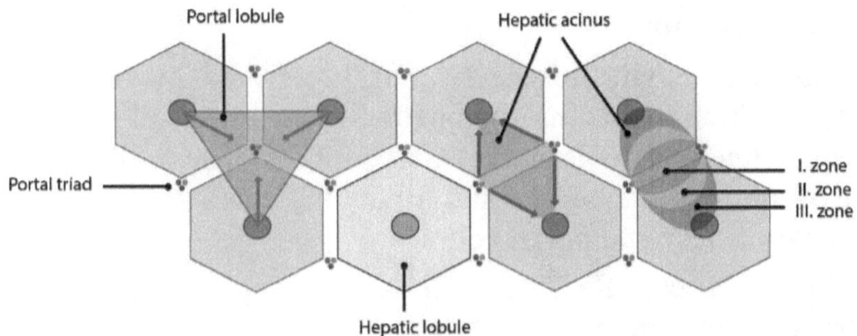

Portal canal: Three structures are found grouped together in the loose connective tissue surrounding the plates of hepatocytes. These include branches of the hepatic artery, the hepatic portal vein (venule) and the intralobular bile ductule. This group of three structures has been called a portal triad but now it is called a portal canal or portal area, because it also contains a fourth structure, the lymphatic vessels and vagus nerve (parasympathetic) fibres.

Arterial Supply and Venous Drainage

The liver has a unique dual blood supply:

Hepatic artery proper (25%) – supplies the structures of the liver with arterial blood. It is derived from the coeliac trunk.

Hepatic portal vein (75%) – supplies the liver with partially deoxygenated blood, carrying nutrients absorbed from the small intestine. This is the dominant blood supply to the liver parenchyma, and allows the liver to perform its gut-related functions, such as detoxification.

Venous drainage of the liver is achieved through hepatic veins. The central veins of the hepatic lobule form collecting veins which then combine to form multiple hepatic veins. These hepatic veins then combine and drain into the inferior vena cava.

Nerve Supply

The parenchyma of the liver is innervated by the hepatic plexus, which contains sympathetic (coeliac plexus) and parasympathetic (vagus nerve) nerve fibres. These fibres enter the liver at the porta hepatis and follow the course of branches of the hepatic artery and portal vein.

Glisson's capsule, the fibrous covering of the liver, is innervated by branches of the lower intercostal nerves. Distension of the capsule results in a sharp, well localised pain.

Lymphatic Drainage

The lymphatic vessels of the anterior aspect of the liver drain into hepatic lymph nodes. These lie along the hepatic vessels and ducts in the lesser omentum, and empty in the colic lymph nodes which in turn, drain into the cisterna chyli.

Lymphatics from the posterior aspect of the liver however, drain into phrenic and posterior mediastinal nodes which join the right lymphatic and thoracic ducts.

Physiology of the Liver

Digestion

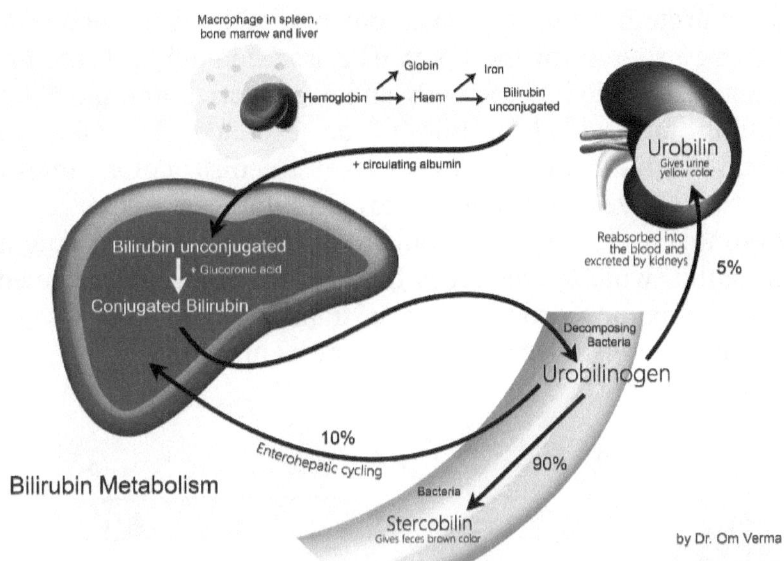

The liver plays an active role in the process of digestion through the production of bile. Bile is a mixture of water, bile salts, cholesterol, the pigment bilirubin, lecithin, and IgA. Hepatocytes in the liver produce bile, which then passes through the bile ducts to be stored in the gallbladder. When food containing fats reaches the duodenum, the cells of the duodenum release the hormone cholecystokinin to stimulate the gallbladder to release bile. Bile travels through the bile ducts and is released into the duodenum where it emulsifies large masses of fat. The emulsification of fats by bile turns the large clumps of fat into smaller pieces that have more surface area and are therefore easier for the body to digest.

Bilirubin present in bile is a product of the liver's digestion of worn out red blood cells. Macrophage cells of spleen and Kupffer cells in the liver catch and destroy old, worn out red blood cells and pass their components on to hepatocytes. Hepatocytes metabolize hemoglobin, the red oxygen-carrying pigment of red blood cells, into the components heme and globin. Globin protein is further broken down to amino acids and used as an energy source for the body. The iron-containing heme group cannot be recycled by the body and is converted into the pigment bilirubin and added to bile to be excreted from the body. Bilirubin gives bile its distinctive greenish color. Intestinal bacteria convert bilirubin into urobilinogen. 90% of this urobilinogen is further converted into a brown pigment stercobilin, which gives feces their brown color and excreted in feces. Remaining urobilinogen is transported to liver by portal vein, half of which is excreted in urine as urobilin.

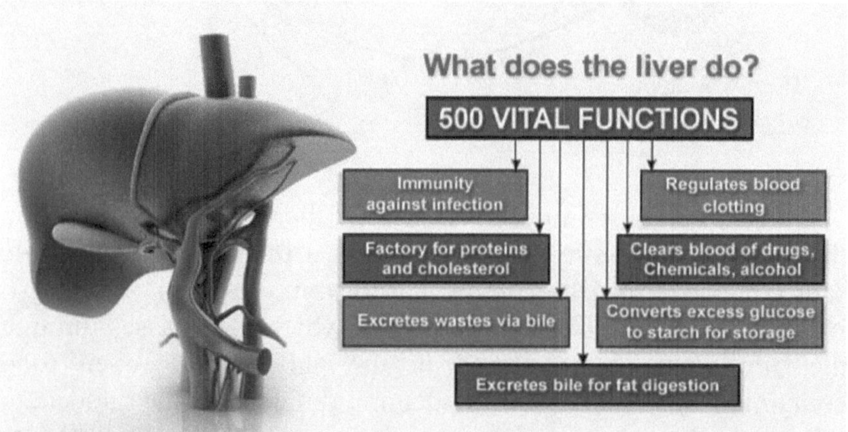

Metabolism

The hepatocytes of the liver are tasked with many of the important metabolic jobs that support the cells of the body. Because all of the blood leaving the digestive system passes through the hepatic portal vein, the liver is responsible for metabolizing carbohydrate, lipids, and proteins into biologically useful materials.

Our digestive system breaks down carbohydrates into the monosaccharide glucose, which cells use as a primary energy source. Blood entering the liver through the hepatic portal vein is extremely rich in glucose from digested food. Hepatocytes absorb much of this glucose and store it as the macromolecule glycogen, a branched polysaccharide that allows the hepatocytes to pack away large amounts of glucose and quickly release glucose between meals. The absorption and release of glucose by the hepatocytes helps to maintain balance and protects the rest of the body from dangerous spikes and drops in the blood glucose level.

Fatty acids in the blood passing through the liver are absorbed by hepatocytes and metabolized to produce energy in the form of ATP. Glycerol, another lipid component, is converted into glucose by hepatocytes through the process of gluconeogenesis. Hepatocytes can also produce lipids like cholesterol, phospholipids, and lipoproteins that are used by other cells throughout the body. Much of the cholesterol produced by hepatocytes gets excreted from the body as a component of bile.

Dietary proteins are broken down into their basic component amino acids by the digestive system before being passed on to the hepatic portal vein. Amino acids entering the liver require metabolic processing before they can be used as an energy source. Hepatocytes first remove the amine groups of the amino acids and convert them into ammonia and eventually urea. Urea is less toxic than ammonia and can be excreted in urine as a waste product of digestion. The remaining parts of the amino acids can be broken down into ATP or converted into new glucose molecules through the process of gluconeogenesis.

Detoxification

As blood from the digestive organs passes through the hepatic portal circulation, the hepatocytes of the liver monitor the contents of the blood and remove many potentially toxic substances before they can reach the rest of the body. Enzymes in hepatocytes metabolize many of these toxins such as alcohol and drugs into their inactive metabolites. And in order to keep hormone levels within homeostatic limits, the liver also metabolizes and removes from circulation hormones produced by the body's own glands.

Storage

The liver provides storage of many essential nutrients, vitamins, and minerals obtained from blood passing through the hepatic portal system. Glucose is transported into hepatocytes under the influence of the hormone insulin and stored as the glycogen. Hepatocytes also absorb and store fatty acids from digested triglycerides. The storage of these nutrients allows the liver to maintain the homeostasis or balance of blood glucose. Our liver also stores vitamins and minerals - such as vitamins A, D, E, K, and B12, and the minerals iron (ferritin) and copper - in order to provide a constant supply of these essential substances to the tissues of the body.

Unfortunately, one common hereditary disorder called hemochromatosis causes the liver to store too much iron, potentially leading to liver disease. Modern DNA health testing can help you find out if you are genetically at higher risk of acquiring this condition or others like Gaucher disease and alpha-1 antitrypsin deficiency, all of which increase your risk of developing liver disease.

Production

Most of plasma proteins except gamma globulins (approximately 15-50 gm/day) are produced in liver. If half of the plasma proteins are lost, it can be replaced within 12 weeks. Albumins and globulins are proteins that maintain the isotonic environment of the blood so that cells of the body do not gain or lose water in the presence of body fluids.

With the exception of factor VIII, the blood clotting factors like prothrombin, fibrinogen, factors II, VII, IX, and X are made exclusively in hepatocytes. Biosynthesis of factors II, VII, IX, and X depends on vitamin K. Prothrombin and fibrinogen and other coagulation factors are involved in the formation of blood clots.

Liver also produce enzymes e.g. transaminases and alkaline phosphatase. Transaminases are important in the synthesis of amino acids, which form proteins. Transaminases include the aspartate aminotransferase (AST) and the alanine aminotransferase (ALT) and are sensitive indicators of liver cell injury and are most helpful in recognizing acute hepatocellular diseases such as hepatitis.

Alkaline phosphatase (ALP) and gamma glutamyl transpeptidase (GGT) activities are usually elevated in cholestasis and obstructive jaundice.

A variety of carrier proteins e.g. transcortin, transferrin, cruloplasmin, haptoglobin and haemopexin are also produced in liver.

Immunity

The liver functions as an organ of the immune system through the function of the Kupffer cells that line the sinusoids. Kupffer cells are a type of fixed macrophage that form part of the mononuclear phagocyte system along with macrophages in the spleen and lymph nodes. Kupffer cells play an important role by capturing and digesting bacteria, fungi, parasites, worn-out blood cells, and cellular debris. The large volume of blood passing through the hepatic portal system and the liver allows Kupffer cells to clean large volumes of blood very quickly.

Liver cancer

Liver cancer is uncommon in the United States but is common worldwide due to risk factors such as chronic hepatitis B and hepatitis C infections and aflatoxin exposure. Symptoms may include jaundice (a yellowing of the skin), pain in the upper abdomen, right shoulder blade pain, and weight loss. Doctors diagnose the condition using a combination of imaging tests and blood tests.

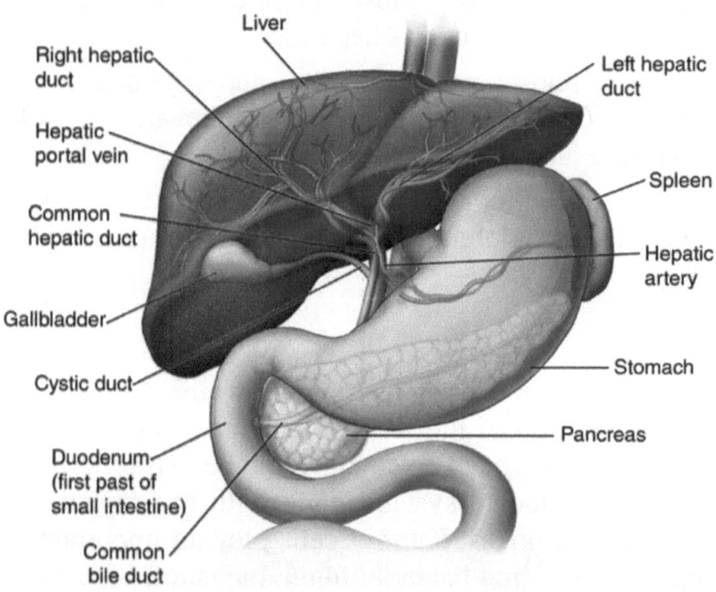

Liver cancer arises in the liver. It's important to distinguish primary liver cancer (hepatocellular carcinoma) and bile duct cancer (cholangiocarcinoma) from metastatic liver cancers which begin in other places of the body and spread to the liver. Liver metastases are much more common than primary liver cancers and are treated in the way that a primary cancer (such as lung cancer or breast cancer) are treated, instead of the way that primary liver cancer is treated.

The functions of the liver are important to know as you look at the possible symptoms of the disease. The liver plays roles in detoxifying substances, secreting bile to aid in digestion of fats and making hormones that are important in the production of red blood cells.

In addition to the cancers mentioned above, there are less common types of liver cancer. A few of these include hepatoblastoma, a rare form of childhood cancer, and angiosarcoma of the liver. We shall focus primarily on primary liver cancer and bile duct cancer.

Incidence

Liver cancer is the sixth common cancer and the second leading cause of death from cancer around the world. It is significantly more observable among male with its highest incidence in the age group of 45 to 60 years.

In the year 2020, an estimated 42,810 adults (30,170 men and 12,640 women) in the United States will be diagnosed with primary liver cancer. Since 1980, incidence of liver cancer has tripled. Between 2007 and 2016, the number of people diagnosed with the disease increased by approximately 2% annually. Men are about 3 times more likely than women to be diagnosed with the disease.

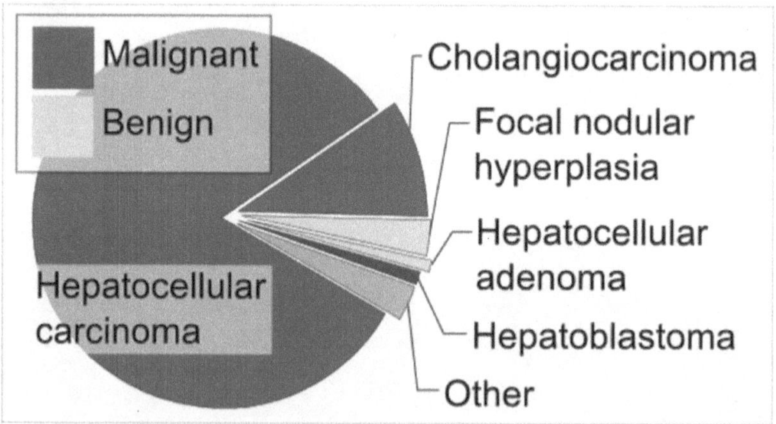

It is estimated that 30,160 deaths (20,020 men and 10,140 women) from this disease will occur in 2020. For men, liver cancer is the fifth most common cause of cancer death. It is the seventh most common cause of cancer death among women. The overall death rate has more than doubled from 1980 to 2017.

When compared with the United States, liver cancer is much more common in sub-Saharan Africa and Southeast Asia. In some countries, it is the most common cancer type.

The 5-year survival rate tells you what percent of people live at least 5 years after the cancer is found. Percent means how many out of 100. The general 5-year survival rate is 18%, compared to just 3% 40 years ago. Survival rates depend on several factors, including the stage of the disease.

For the 44% of people who are diagnosed at an early stage, the 5-year survival rate is 33%. If liver cancer has spread to surrounding tissues or organs and/or the regional lymph nodes, the 5-year survival rate is 11%. If the cancer has spread to a distant part of the body, the 5-year survival rate is 2%. However, even if the cancer is found at a more advanced stage, treatments are available that help many people with liver cancer experience a quality of life similar to that of before their diagnosis, at least for some time. If surgery is possible, that generally results in higher survival rates across all stages of the disease, but I am doubtful.

Cause

We don't know the precise causes of liver cancer, but some of the risk factors include excessive alcohol use, smoking, liver infections such as hepatitis B and hepatitis C, certain other medical and genetic conditions, and other concerns.

Liver cancer can affect both children and adults but occurs most often in adults. There are several types of liver cancer, but the risk factors below refer to adult primary liver cancer, called hepatocellular carcinoma and bile duct cancer (cholangio-carcinoma). Studies have found that liver cancer and bile duct cancer are increasing worldwide, and are the leading cause of cancer deaths in some regions.

There is no screening test for liver cancer, but being aware of your risk factors and knowing the signs and symptoms can help detect it when it's still in early, and more treatable, stages.

Common Risk Factors

Cancer begins when a series of gene mutations lead a cell to grow out of control. How this happens in liver cancer isn't confirmed, but several mechanisms have been postulated. What is known is that several factors increase one's risk of developing the disease. Some of them do so substantially, whereas others may raise the risk only a small amount. There are other risk factors that are considered, though experts aren't sure if they are indeed related.

Having a risk factor for liver cancer does not mean that you will develop the disease. It's also possible to get liver cancer even if you don't have any known risk factors.

It is usually a combination of factors working together that result in the development of a tumor. Combinations of risk factors can be additive, but can also be multiplicative, such as with the combinations of alcohol and smoking or hepatitis B and smoking.

Race and Sex

Asians and Pacific Islanders develop liver cancer more often than people of other races, largely due to the hepatitis epidemic among these regions. Caucasians develop liver cancer less frequently, but the disease appears to be increasing.

Liver cancer is more common in men than women, although the reasons aren't entirely clear.

Hepatitis B Infection

Chronic hepatitis B infection is a major risk factor for the development of liver cancer and is the leading cause of this cancer in Africa and most of Asia. People with chronic hepatitis B are at risk for the development of liver cancer, though some people with chronic hepatitis B are at more risk than others.

Hepatitis treatments are available, but many people are not aware they carry the virus or live in an area in which medical care is less than optimal. Overall, hepatitis B carriers are 100 times more likely to develop liver cancer, and 2.5 percent of people with cirrhosis due to hepatitis B (and 0.5 to 1 percent of people without cirrhosis) will develop the disease each year.

While 95% of people with hepatitis B clear the virus, but after infection roughly 5% will become chronic carriers.

Hepatitis C Infection

Hepatitis C is also a major risk factor for the development of liver cancer and is currently the leading cause of liver cancer in the United States, Europe, and Japan. Unlike hepatitis B, many people do not clear the virus, and it becomes a progressive disease. Roughly 20 to 30 percent of people who are infected go on to develop cirrhosis.

When hepatitis C is found and treated with antiviral medications, the risk of cirrhosis, and likely liver cancer can be greatly reduced.

Most people with hepatitis C are unaware they are infected. Therefore, it's recommended that all American adults born between 1945 and 1965 get tested.

Non-Alcoholic Fatty Liver Disease (NAFLD)

Non-alcoholic fatty liver disease is a condition similar to alcoholic liver disease, but it results in an accumulation of fat in the liver (fatty liver) by a different mechanism. It's thought to be an autoimmune disease (in which the body makes antibodies against itself) and may have a genetic component.

With NAFLD, the risk of liver cancer is increased. Closely related, metabolic syndrome may also be a risk factor for liver cancer.

Immunosuppression

Immunosuppression increases the risk of liver cancer, as well as other cancers. Organ transplant recipients are twice as likely to develop liver cancer as the general population, and the risk is even higher for those who have received a liver transplant.

Having HIV/AIDS is associated with a five-fold greater risk of developing liver cancer.

Lupus (Systemic Lupus Erythematosus)

The reason is uncertain, but people who have lupus are more than twice as likely to develop liver cancer.

Diabetes

People who have diabetes have a risk of liver cancer two to three times higher than the general population. Of interest, it appears that the diabetic medication Glucophage (metformin) may reduce this risk.

Chemical Exposures (and Occupational Risk)

A number of chemical exposures have been linked to the development of liver cancer and are probable carcinogens.

One exposure that the general public may encounter is arsenic in well water.

Occupational exposures are also of concern, including exposure to vinyl chloride (found in plastics), acrylamide, PFOA or perfluorooctanoic acid (found in dry cleaning methods), polychlorinated biphenyls (PCBs), perfluorinated chemicals (PFCs), benzo(a)pyrene (BaP), and trichloroethylene.

Sclerosing Cholangitis

Sclerosing cholangitis is a chronic liver disease associated with inflammatory bowel disease (such as Crohn's disease that involves the colon and ulcerative colitis).

Sclerosing cholangitis causes inflammation and scarring of the bile ducts such that bile backs up into the liver causing scarring there as well.

Approximately 10-15% of people with sclerosing cholangitis develop cholangiocarcinoma (bile duct cancer).

Aflatoxin Exposure

Though an uncommon risk factor in the United States, this is a more significant one worldwide. Aflatoxin B1 is a toxin produced by fungi (of the genus Aspergillus) that grows on foods such as wheat, peanuts, other groundnuts, soybeans, and corn. The toxin causes damage to the p53 gene in liver cells—a tumor suppressor gene that helps repair damaged DNA and inhibit the growth of harmful cells.

Research is ongoing and studies are exploring whether aflatoxin causes liver cancer on its own or as a co-factor when combined with hepatitis B.

Strict food regulations and testing make exposure uncommon in the United States, through exposure and poisoning are common worldwide. The toxin is often found in foods that have not been stored properly, usually in warm and tropical climates. American travelers to such areas likely should not worry, though—it's thought that long-term exposure is required to cause liver cancer.

Genetics

Liver cancer can run in families (even without a known genetic disease), and having a relative with the disease (on either side) increases your risk. The risk is greatest when it is a first degree relative such as a parent, sibling, or child.

Hemochromatosis

Hereditary hemochromatosis (iron overload disease) is a condition marked by the body's increased absorption and storage of iron, often in the liver. In time, the condition usually leads to cirrhosis and eventually liver failure (as well as other medical problems).

The risk of liver cancer in people who have hemochromatosis is 20 times higher than that of the general population.

Treatment (periodically withdrawing blood) can reduce the risk of problems, but many people are unaware they have the condition until they develop problems. It's thought that 1 million people in the United States are affected by one of the types of hemochromatosis.

Primary Biliary Cirrhosis

Primary biliary cirrhosis is a condition that appears to have a genetic component, as it runs in families. It is a progressive, autoimmune disease in which bile builds up in the liver, damaging bile ducts and leading to liver damage and cirrhosis.

Primary biliary cirrhosis is associated with a high risk of liver carcinoma, similar to that found in people with chronic hepatitis C.

Wilson's Disease

Wilson's disease is a rare genetic disorder characterized by the accumulation of copper in the body and is thought to be a risk factor for liver cancer.

Other Hereditary Diseases

Other hereditary diseases that may increase the risk of liver cancer include alpha-1 antitrypsin deficiency, tyrosinemia, acute hepatic porphyrias, porphyria cutanea tarda, and glycogen storage disease.

Lifestyle Risk Factors

Lifestyle factors are important in the development of liver cancer. While you cannot control many of the common risk factors mentioned above, you do have the ability to influence these.

Excessive, Long-Term Alcohol Use

Excessive, long-term use of alcohol can cause a number of liver diseases, including alcoholic hepatitis and alcoholic liver disease. Over time, cirrhosis develops with marked scarring of the liver, and often, liver failure.

Liver cancer is primarily associated with heavy drinking, or the intake of more than three drinks on a daily basis, though lesser amounts can still cause significant and irreversible liver disease.

Smoking

Smoking is a risk factor for many cancers, and liver cancer is no exception. Several studies suggest a link between smoking and liver cancer, and those who both smoke and drink heavily have a significantly greater risk of the disease.

Children who are born to parents who smoked either before or during pregnancy are at an increased risk of a rare type of liver cancer called hepatoblastoma.

Obesity

The role of obesity in liver cancer is uncertain by itself, but obesity does increase the risk of developing non-alcoholic liver disease, a condition that quadruples the risk of liver cancer, as well as diabetes, which is associated with triple the risk.

Anabolic Steroid Use

Anabolic steroids, such as those used by weightlifters, are a risk factor for liver disease and liver cancer.

Chewing Betel Quid

Uncommon in the United States, chewing betel quid is a risk factor for liver cancer in regions where this is commonly practiced.

Other Risk Factors

There is some evidence that gallbladder removal (cholecystectomy) increases risk, though researchers are not certain of the connection. There is a confusion whether there is an increased risk related to current use of birth control pills.

There may be some risk related to medical radiation (such as CT scans of the abdomen), but this risk is likely largely outweighed by the benefits of these tests.

The parasite that causes schistosomiasis (highly endemic in Egypt) has been studied for its possible role in liver cancer. Instead of being a risk factor, it's thought that it is a co-factor in liver cancer related to hepatitis B and C infections.

Autoimmune hepatitis and gallstones are also risk factors for liver cancer.

Symptoms of Liver Cancer

The signs and symptoms of liver cancer are most often the result of liver damage and may include yellowing of the skin (jaundice), right-sided abdominal or shoulder blade pain, or a lump in the right upper abdomen. However, many of the warning signs are non-specific, such as weight loss and fatigue.

Sometimes the complications of liver cancer, such as a bile duct obstruction, anemia, or bleeding are the first symptoms. *Since there's no screening test for liver cancer, having an awareness of the potential signs and symptoms is the only way to find the disease early.*

It's important to briefly differentiate primary liver cancer—that which originates in the liver—from liver metastases, which is the spread of cancer (breast or lung, for example) from another region of the body to the liver. Liver cancer is usually a single large tumor, while metastases (spread) are usually small and multiple.

Primary liver cancer usually causes symptoms relatively early, whereas liver metastases (which are much more common) may occupy a significant part of the liver before they are detected. Symptoms are similar for hepatocellular carcinoma (liver cancer) and cholangiocarcinoma (bile duct cancer), but bile duct cancers tend to cause symptoms of obstruction (such as jaundice) earlier than many liver cancers.

Like many types of cancer, liver cancer usually has very few symptoms or signs in the early stages of the disease. As the disease progresses, its symptoms begin to show up slowly, prompting one to seek medical attention. Due to this delayed onset of symptoms, liver cancer is often diagnosed in an advanced stage (unless the tumor originates near a bile duct and causes an obstruction early).

An Abdominal Mass or Lump

You may feel a very hard lump or swelling in the region just below your rib cage on your right side. Often, this mass is painless, and if you have pain, you may feel more discomfort in the areas surrounding the mass. Sometimes liver cancer causes enlargement of the spleen as well, which can result in pain or a mass felt in the left upper abdomen.

Right-Sided Abdominal Pain

Pain, discomfort, or aching on the right side of the abdomen just under the ribs may occur due to the pressure of a liver tumor on other structures or nerves in this region. Take in a deep breath and press lightly upward under your rib cage on the right side—this is 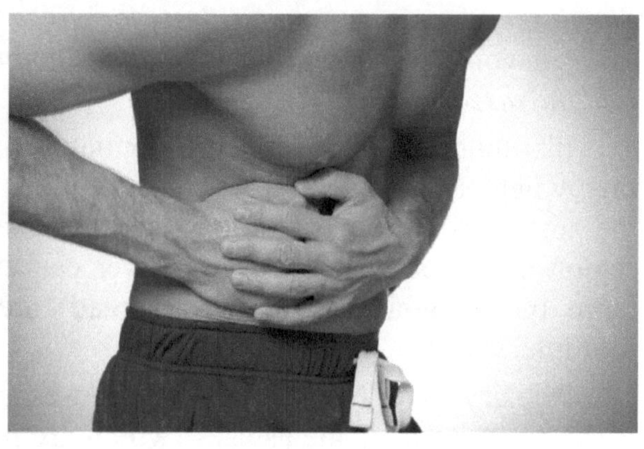 roughly where your liver lies. If you have an enlarged liver due to any reason, the edge of your liver may be felt lower in your abdomen.

Right Shoulder-Blade Pain

Shoulder-blade pain can be a symptom, because the tumor (or spread from the tumor) can irritate nerves that tell your brain the pain is coming from your shoulder blade when it's actually coming from the liver. This pain is typically felt in the right shoulder, though it may occur on either side. The pain may also extend into your back. If you experience this, especially if you haven't engaged in any recent physical activity that might explain it, see your physician.

Jaundice

Jaundice refers to a condition in which the skin, as well as the white part of the eyes, appears yellow. It is caused by the build-up of bilirubin in the skin.

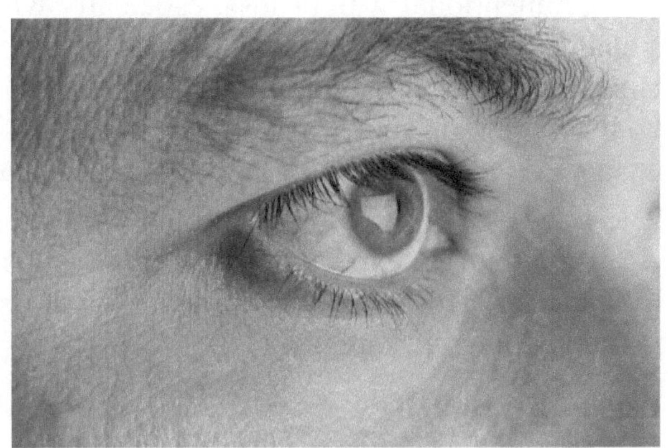

It is more easily detected in natural light, such as being outside, than in indoor light. In addition to yellowing of the skin, some people notice that their stool appear pale and whitish instead of brown. At the same time, urine may appear darker than normal, even without dehydration.

Itching

The build-up of bile salts in the skin, which results in jaundice, can also cause itching. We don't often think of itching as a serious symptom, but the itching associated with liver dysfunction can be very intense.

Bloat and Shortness of Breath

Fluid collection in the abdomen is known as ascites, can indicate liver cancer. It may feel like bloating at first; some people note that their clothes don't fit properly in the waistline or their belt size changes even though they haven't gained weight. In time, fluid build-up in the abdomen can push upward on the lungs causing shortness of breath.

Unintentional Weight Loss or Gain

Unintentional weight loss, especially when it's not related to a change in diet or exercise, it always deserves a visit to a doctor. Unexplained weight loss is defined as the loss of 5 percent of body weight or more over a six to 12 month period without trying. An example would be a 200 pound man losing 10 pounds over a period of six months without a change in habits.

Rapid and unexpected weight gain is also a possible sign of liver cancer. This usually occurs due to the rapid build-up of fluid in the abdomen (ascites).

Loss of Appetite

A loss of appetite may occur with many disorders, but can be quite profound with liver problems. This may be accompanied by a sense of becoming full very rapidly, even when eating only small meals. As these symptoms could be warning signs of not only liver cancer but other cancers, you should visit your physician.

Nausea and Vomiting

There are several reasons why liver cancer can lead to nausea and vomiting, and this is a common symptom at all stages of the disease. There are a vast number of causes for nausea

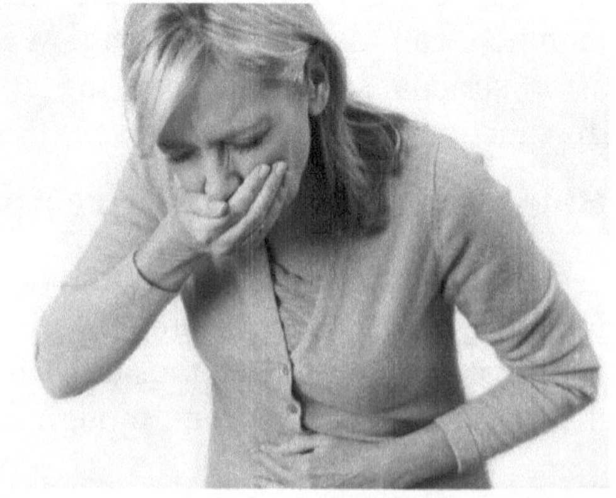

and vomiting, but when it occurs frequently, or if it is worsening, talk to your doctor.

Fatigue and/or Weakness

It seems everyone is tired these days, but cancer-related fatigue often takes things to a new level. Cancer fatigue is different from ordinary tiredness, and it is not the kind of fatigue that improves with a good night of sleep. Sometimes this symptom is easier to see if you look back at a period of six to 12 months and gauge your energy today against what it was at that time.

Fever

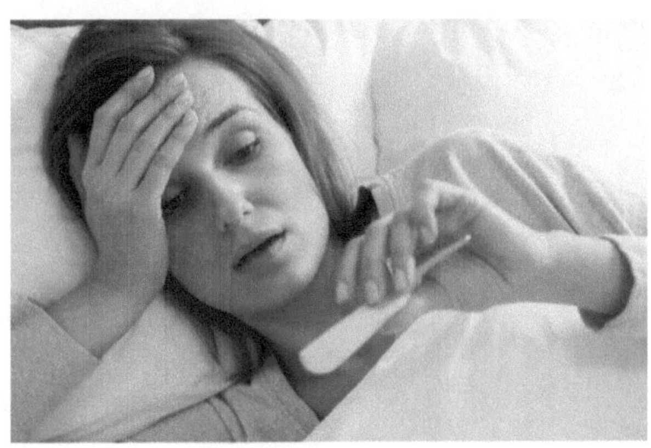

A low-grade, but persistent fever, something physicians refer to as a "fever of unknown origin" or FUO, is a fairly common symptom of liver cancer. An FUO is defined as a temperature greater than 101 degrees that last for three or more weeks and that cannot be tied to an obvious cause after three or more doctor's visits (or three days in the hospital). There are several other potential causes of a persistent fever, but having one is a good reason to see your physician.

General Feeling of Being Unwell

If you have a general sense that you are not well, see your doctor. Sometimes, symptoms can be hard to define in terms like those listed above. Our bodies often do a good job of "telling" us when something is wrong if we only take the time to listen.

Rare Symptoms

Some liver cancers secrete hormones that can cause additional symptoms. These may include low blood sugar (hypoglycemia) that can result in lightheadedness and fainting, especially in people who haven't eaten for a while; breast enlargement (gynecomastia); testicular atrophy; and a high red blood cell count.

Complications

Liver cancer can result in a number of complications. They may result from the pressure of a tumor on the bile duct or other organs, hormones produced by the cancer cells, liver dysfunction that results in the build-up of toxins in the body, or other mechanisms.

Some potential complications include:

Anemia

Anemia, a low red blood cell count, is a very common complication of liver cancer and may appear due to a few mechanisms, including a lack of clotting factors in the blood leading to bleeding. Anemia can be insidious at first, and it frequently causes symptoms such as fatigue, shortness of breath, a rapid heart rate, pale skin, and lightheadedness. Since liver cancer can sometimes result in erythrocytosis (increased red blood cell production) as well, these effects sometimes cancel each other out.

Bile Duct Obstruction

Bile is produced in the liver. Several ducts ensure that it gets transported to the small intestine, either via the gallbladder or directly. Liver tumors or bile duct tumors can grow within a duct or exert pressure near one, resulting in bile duct obstruction.

When a duct is obstructed for either reason, it usually results in the rapid onset of severe and constant pain in the right upper abdomen, nausea, vomiting, jaundice, and itching.

Bleeding

The liver is responsible for making proteins (clotting factors) that help your blood clot. When a large percentage of your liver has been overtaken by cancer, these factors are no longer produced in sufficient numbers. The result is that bleeding may occur (even with a normal number of platelets) and anemia may ensue. The first sign is often bleeding when you brush your teeth or frequent nosebleeds. More serious bleeding, such as internal hemorrhage, may occur when the cancer is advanced.

Portal Hypertension

Liver cancer (and other liver diseases like cirrosis) can lead to bleeding from the digestive tract in another way as well. A tumor within the liver can make it difficult for blood to flow through the small veins in the organ that lead to the large portal vein. The resulting pressure on the vein (portal hypertension) causes increased pressure in blood vessels upstream, such as those in the esophagus.

These veins are weaker than the larger portal vein and can develop into varicose veins, much like you see on people's legs, or on the abdomen at times with liver disease. When these varicosities rupture, it can result in massive bleeding into the esophagus (esophageal variceal 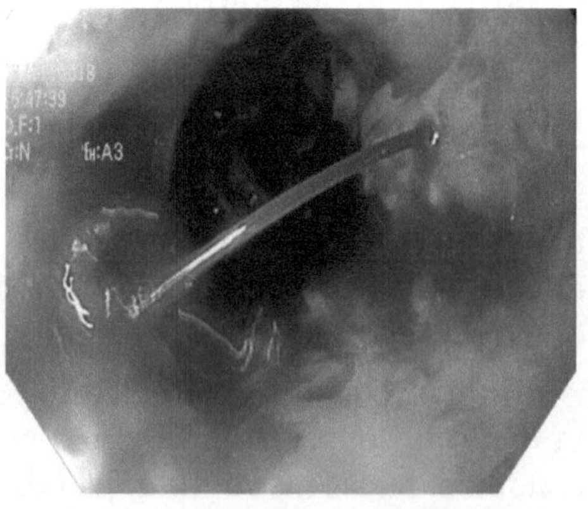 bleeding, which can be life-threatening if not treated promptly. Bleeding may occur in the stomach and intestines as well due to the same mechanism.

High Blood Calcium (Hypercalcemia)

Liver cancer may result in a high calcium level in the blood (hypercalcemia of malignancy) through a few different mechanisms. This may cause nausea and vomiting, extreme muscle weakness, and confusion, which can progress to coma and even death if not treated.

Hepatorenal Syndrome

Hepatorenal syndrome is a condition in which liver disease leads to kidney disease due to changes in blood vessels and reduced blood flow to the kidneys. Hepatorenal syndrome is very common with liver cancer and other forms of liver disease, and it's estimated that 40 percent of people who have cirrhosis will develop the syndrome within five years. Unfortunately, it is usually irreversible in these individuals unless liver transplantation is performed.

Hepatic Encephalopathy

Hepatic encephalopathy can be a frightening complication of liver cancer but is actually a reversible cause of symptoms that can look like Alzheimer's disease.

Toxins that the liver is unable to remove travel to the brain. This can result in memory loss, disorientation, personality changes, and severe confusion. Symptoms may begin mildly with difficulty doing math-centered tasks, like balancing a checkbook. Other symptoms may include breath that has a sweet odor and flapping of the arms when they are held out straight in front of a person. There are ways to treat the encephalopathy, but the prognosis usually depends on the extent of the tumor.

When to See a Doctor

If you note any of the signs and symptoms above or any you can't explain, see your doctor. While many can indicate harmless conditions, if liver cancer is present, the prognosis is generally better the earlier the disease is diagnosed. People who have no risk factors for liver cancer can and do develop the disease at times—something worth keeping in mind if you're unsure about speaking with your physician.

If you do have risk factors for liver cancer, such as cirrhosis, your situation is a bit more challenging. You may already be experiencing similar symptoms as a result of an existing health issue. In this case, the key point is to watch for a change in your symptoms.

One study found that symptoms that alerted physicians to the presence of liver cancer in people with chronic liver disease included right upper quadrant pain, enlargement of the liver (cirrhosis usually causes it to shrink), more fatigue, a change in mood, worsening of portal hypertension, hemorrhoids, bleeding, and diabetes that had become difficult to control. If you notice any of these symptoms, contact your doctor right away.

Diagnosis

Primary liver cancer (also called hepatocellular carcinoma) occurs when abnormal cells in the liver begin to grow uncontrollably. Generally speaking, the diagnosis of liver cancer involves the following steps—a physical examination, blood tests, imaging and sometimes a biopsy.

Depending on whether or not you have been previously diagnosed with chronic liver disease and/or cirrhosis, which is when the liver irreversibly scars as a result of chronic liver disease, your doctor may proceed a bit differently with diagnosing liver cancer.

Because the outcome in patients with advanced HCC is uniformly dismal, early diagnosis is crucial in order to provide effective treatment. Consequently, routine screening for HCC is recommended in patients with cirrhosis from any cause; some guidelines also recommend testing in other patients at high risk. Screening is typically performed using ultrasonography (US), with or without serum alpha-fetoprotein (AFP) measurement, generally every 6 months.

Physical Examination

After reviewing your risk factors for liver cancer (for example, whether you have a history of cirrhosis or a history of alcohol abuse), if your doctor is suspicious for cancer, he will pay close attention to your abdomen, especially the right side where your liver is located. More specifically, your doctor will press beneath your right ribcage in order to determine if your liver is enlarged.

Your doctor will also look for other signs of long-term liver disease (which increase your risk of having liver cancer) like:

- An enlarged spleen, located in the upper left side of your abdomen
- Visible veins on your abdomen
- A fluid-filled, swollen abdomen Ascites
- Evidence of jaundice (for example, yellowing of the white part of your eye

Labs

There are a number of blood tests your doctor may order to help diagnose liver cancer and determine the potential cause of the cancer:

- **Complete blood cell count (CBC)** - WBC count, WBC differential), (RBC) count, Hematocrit (packed cell volume), Hemoglobin, Red blood cell indices, Platelet count & Mean platelet volume

- **Electrolyte levels**

- **Liver function tests (LFTs)** - These tests include prothrombin time (PT/INR), Total Proteins, albumin, bilirubin (direct and indirect), SGOT, SGPT, Alkaline phosphatase and others.

- Coagulation studies (e.g., international normalized ratio [INR], Prothrombin Time, partial thromboplastin time [PTT])

Alpha-Fetoprotein (AFP) Tumor Marker

AFP is a protein that is high in fetuses but falls to low levels after birth. AFP levels may be elevated because of production by the tumor or by regenerating hepatocytes. Therefore, AFP levels are also frequently elevated in chronic active hepatitis C (levels of 200-300 ng/mL are not uncommon), but in those patients the levels tend to fluctuate and do not progressively increase. AFP levels can also be elevated because of other conditions, such as following liver resection (transient until regeneration complete), recovery following toxic injury, or seroconversion following hepatitis B infection (typically inducing transient exacerbation of inflammation).

When elevated, the AFP is 75-91% specific, and values greater than 400 ng/mL are generally considered diagnostic of HCC in the proper clinical context, including appropriate radiologic findings. Better biologic markers, including AFP variants, are being investigated.

Cirrhosis Tests

If a physical exam or imaging test reveals that you have chronic liver disease and/or cirrhosis, but the cause behind it has not yet been determined, your doctor will order a series of blood tests. For instance, he will order blood tests to check for infection with hepatitis B and C. He will also likely order ferritin and iron levels to check for hemochromatosis, another common cause of cirrhosis.

Liver Function Tests (LFTs)

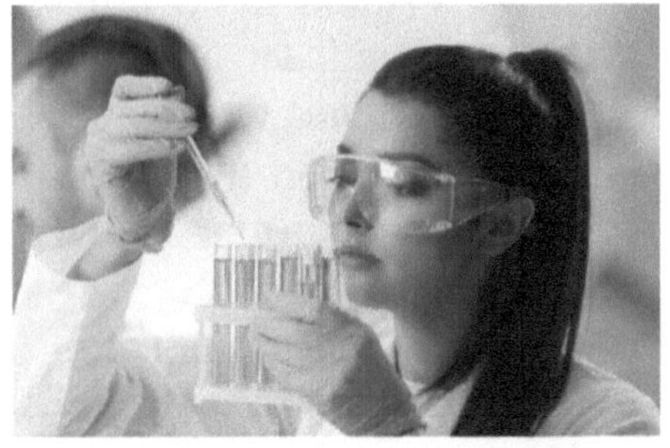

LFTs comprise a series of blood tests that give your doctors an idea of how well your liver is functioning. These tests can also help your doctor figure out the best treatment plan for your liver cancer. For instance, if your liver cancer is small and contained and your liver appears to be working well, then removing the cancer by surgery may be a sensible option.

Other Tests

Your doctor may order other blood tests to determine how well other organs in your body are working. For example, he may order blood tests that evaluate how well your kidneys are working. Additionally, since liver cancer may impact blood levels of glucose, calcium, and platelets, these tests may also be ordered.

Laboratory results suggestive or indicative of disease severity include the following:

- **Anemia -** Low hemoglobin may be related to bleeding from varices or other sources
- **Thrombocytopenia -** A platelet count below 100,000/μL is highly suggestive of significant portal hypertension/splenomegaly
- **Hyponatremia** is commonly found in patients with cirrhosis and ascites and may be a marker of advanced liver disease
- Increased serum creatinine level may reflect intrinsic renal disease or hepatorenal syndrome
- **Prolonged prothrombin time** (PT)/INR reflects significant impairment of hepatic function that may preclude resection
- **Elevated liver enzymes** SGOP, SGPT reflect active hepatitis due to viral infection, current alcohol use, or other causes
- **Increased bilirubin level** usually indicates jaundice in a advanced liver disease
- **Hypoglycemia** may represent end-stage liver disease (no glycogen stores)

Laboratory findings associated with particular disease etiologies include the following:

- **Hepatitis B surface antigen (HBsAg)/hepatitis B core antibody (anti-HBc), anti-HCV** - Viral hepatitis (current/past)
- **Increased iron saturation** (> 50%) - Underlying hemochromatosis

- **Low α1-antitrypsin levels** - α1-Antitrypsin deficiency
- **Increased AFP** - Levels higher than 400 ng/mL are considered diagnostic with appropriate imaging studies
- **Hypercalcemia** - Ectopic parathyroid hormone production is possible in 5-10% of patients with HCC

Imaging

Imaging tests are essential to diagnosing liver cancer.

Ultrasound

The first test a person may undergo is an ultrasound. During an ultrasound, a probe will be gently pressed on your abdomen to see if there are any masses located in your liver.

CT Scans and MRIs

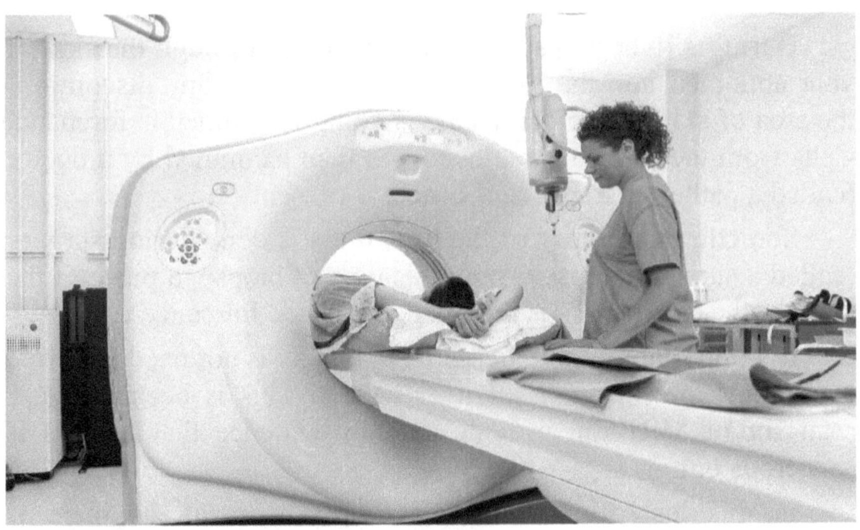

If a mass is seen on an ultrasound, a more sophisticated test like a computed tomography (CT scan) and/or magnetic resonance imaging (MRI) of the liver is done to give more detailed information about the mass, such as:

- Size
- Location in the liver
- Spread to nearby blood vessels or other parts of the abdomen

These imaging tests may also give information about what type of mass is present, meaning whether the mass is benign (non-cancerous) or malignant (cancerous).

Angiography

Lastly, a CT angiography or MRI angiography may be performed to provide a picture of the arteries supplying blood to the liver. For this test, you will need an IV placed in your arm so that contrast dye can be administered during the CT scan or MRI.

Biopsy

During a liver biopsy, a needle is placed through the skin of your abdomen into the liver mass. To minimize any discomfort, the area of skin where the needle is going is numbed beforehand. Cells from the mass are removed and then examined by a doctor (called a pathologist) to see if cancer is present.

Sometimes a biopsy of the liver mass is done during surgery (called a surgical biopsy). With this type of biopsy, a piece of the mass or the entire mass is removed and tested for cancer.

It's important to note that often a biopsy is not needed to rule in (or out) the diagnosis of liver cancer. This is because a CT scan and/or MRI can provide enough evidence that a mass is cancerous or not.

In this instance, avoiding a biopsy is ideal, as there is concern that removing cancerous cells from a mass may "seed" nearby areas with cancer. In that case, a spread of cancer may make a person ineligible for a liver transplant (a potential treatment option).

Regardless, sometimes a biopsy is necessary in order to make the diagnosis if imaging is not conclusive.

Differential Diagnosis

It's important to mention that a cancerous lesion in the liver may not be primary liver cancer but rather a metastatic lesion from another cancer. For example, colon cancer that spreads to the liver is called metastatic colon cancer or secondary liver cancer. In this case, your doctor will need to investigate what the primary cancer is, if not known.

Furthermore, know that there are many potential diagnoses for a liver mass, meaning it's not necessarily cancer.

Two examples of benign (non-cancerous) causes of liver masses include:

Hepatic Hemangioma

Hepatic hemangioma is a mass of blood vessels that is the most common type of benign liver mass. It does not usually cause symptoms, but may cause abdominal discomfort, bloating, or early satiety if it becomes large enough. While a hepatic hemangioma does not usually require treatment, it may need to be removed by a surgeon if it breaks open and bleeds, although this is rare.

Hepatic Adenoma

A hepatic adenoma is a benign liver tumor that usually causes no symptoms unless it bleeds or grows large enough. In a small percentage of cases, a hepatic adenoma may turn into liver cancer, which is why it's generally removed.

Stages of liver cancer

Making an educated treatment decision begins with determining the stage, or progression, of the disease. The stage of liver cancer is one of the most important factors in evaluating treatment options.

Our cancer doctors use a variety of diagnostic tests to evaluate liver cancer and develop an individualized treatment plan. If you have been recently diagnosed, we will review your pathology to confirm you have received the correct diagnosis and staging information and develop a personalized treatment plan. If you have a recurrence, we will perform comprehensive testing and identify a treatment approach that is suited to your needs.

The American Joint Committee on Cancer developed TNM system, the most widely accepted method for liver cancer staging. This system bases the staging criteria on the evaluation of three primary factors:

- **T (tumor):** This describes the number and size of the original tumor.

- **N (node):** This indicates whether the cancer is present in the regional (nearby) lymph nodes.

- **M (metastasis):** This refers to whether cancer has spread to distant parts of the body. (The most common sites of liver cancer spread are the lungs and bones.)

A number (0-4) or the letter X is assigned to each factor. A higher number indicates increasing severity. For instance, a T1 score indicates a smaller tumor than a T2 score. The letter X means the information could not be assessed. Once the T, N and M scores have been assigned, an overall liver cancer stage is assigned.

Unlike other cancers, liver cancer is complicated by the fact that most patients have liver damage that limits the function of the liver. The liver provides important functions for the body, aiding in digesting and detoxification. Reduced liver function may result in severe, even life-threatening conditions. Reduced liver function may also have implications when choosing treatment options.

Several other liver cancer staging systems have been developed that take into account how the function of the liver may affect the prognosis:

- The Barcelona-Clinic Liver Cancer (BCLC) system
- The Cancer of the Liver Italian Program (CLIP) system
- The Okuda system

The Child-Pugh score is part of the BCLC and CLIP staging systems and gives the measure of liver function in people with cirrhosis. The system looks at five factors including levels of bilirubin and albumin in the blood, prothrombin time, accumulation of fluid (ascites) in the abdomen, and impact of liver disease on brain function.

Patients with normal liver function are classified as class A; those with mild abnormalities are class B; and those with severe abnormalities are class C. Liver cancer patients with class C cirrhosis are generally not fit to receive treatment.

Stage I (stage 1 liver cancer): The single primary tumor (any size) has not grown into any blood vessels. The cancer has not spread to nearby lymph nodes or distant sites.

Stage II (stage 2 liver cancer): A single primary tumor (any size) has grown into the blood vessels, or several small tumors are present, all less than five centimeters (two inches) in diameter. The cancer has not spread to nearby lymph nodes or distant sites.

Stage III (stage 3 liver cancer): This stage has three subcategories:

- o **Stage IIIA:** Several tumors have been found, and at least one is larger than five centimeters. The cancer has not spread to nearby lymph nodes or distant sites.

- o **Stage IIIB:** Several tumors have been found, and at least one tumor is growing into a branch of the portal vein or the hepatic vein. The liver cancer has not spread to nearby lymph nodes or distant sites.

- o **Stage IIIC:** The tumor has grown into a nearby organ (other than the gallbladder), or the tumor has grown into the outer covering of the liver. The cancer has not spread to nearby lymph nodes or distant sites.

Stage IV (stage 4 liver cancer): The cancer has spread to nearby lymph nodes and may have grown into nearby blood vessels or organs. Advanced liver cancer does not often metastasize (or travel to distant organs), but when it does, it is most likely to spread to the lungs and bones. Stage IV liver cancer may be:

- o Any T, N1 and M0, meaning the cancer consists of any number or size of tumors in the liver, and it has spread to nearby lymph nodes, but no evidence has been found that the cancer has spread to distant organs or tissue.

- o Any T, any N and M1, meaning the cancer consists of any number or size of tumors in the liver, the cancer may or may not have grown into the lymph nodes, and it has spread to another part of the body.

Treatment

Treatment of hepatocellular carcinoma varies by the stage of disease, a person's likelihood to tolerate surgery, and availability of liver transplant:

Curative intention: for limited disease, when the cancer is limited to one or more areas of within the liver, surgically removing the malignant cells may be curative. This may be accomplished by resection the affected portion of the liver (partial hepatectomy) or in some cases by orthotopic liver transplantation of the entire organ.

"Bridging" intention: for limited disease which qualifies for potential liver transplantation, the person may undergo targeted treatment of some or all of the known tumor while waiting for a donor organ to become available.

"Downstaging" intention: for moderately advanced disease which has not spread beyond the liver, but is too advanced to qualify for curative treatment. The person may be treated by targeted therapies in order to reduce the size or number of active tumors, with the goal of once again qualifying for liver transplant after this treatment.

Palliative intention: for more advanced disease, including spread of cancer beyond the liver or in persons who may not tolerate surgery, treatment intended to decrease symptoms of disease and maximize duration of survival.

Loco-regional therapy (also referred to as liver-directed therapy) refers to any one of several minimally-invasive treatment techniques to focally target the tumor within the liver. These procedures are alternatives to surgery, and may be considered in combination with other strategies, such as a later liver transplantation. Generally, these treatment procedures are performed by interventional radiologists or surgeons, in coordination with a medical oncologist. Loco-regional therapy may refer to either percutaneous therapies (e.g. cryoablation), or arterial catheter-based therapies (chemoembolization or radioembolization).

Surgical resection

Surgical removal of the tumor is associated with better cancer prognosis, but only 5–15% of patients are suitable for surgical resection due to the extent of disease or poor liver function. Surgery is only considered if the entire tumor can be safely removed while preserving sufficient functional liver to maintain normal physiology. Thus, preoperative imaging assessment is critical to determine both the extent of tumor and to estimate the amount of residual liver remaining after surgery. To maintain liver function, residual liver volume should exceed 25% of total liver volume in a non-cirrhotic liver, greater than 40% in a cirrhotic liver. Surgery on diseased or cirrhotic livers is generally associated with higher morbidity and mortality. The overall recurrence rate after resection is 50-60%. The Singapore Liver Cancer Recurrence score can be used to estimate risk of recurrence after surgery.

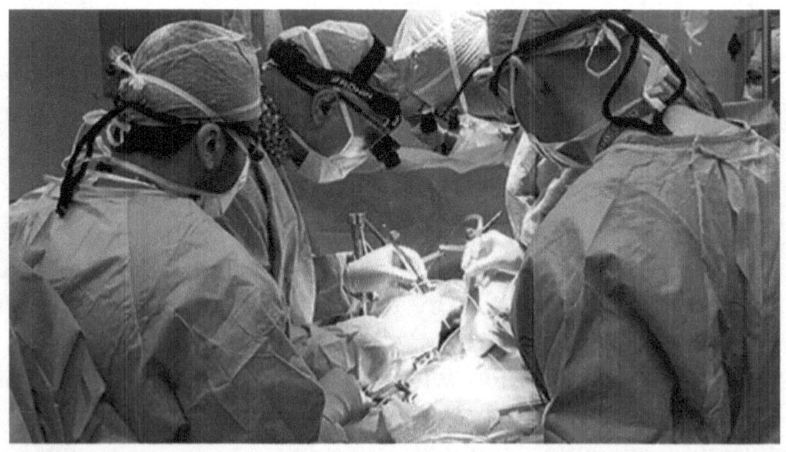

Possible Side Effects

Surgical removal of liver cancer is a major surgery, especially since the liver is rich in blood vessels. This makes bleeding during surgery a major concern.

Other potential side effects of surgery include:

- Infection
- Blood clots
- Complications related to anesthesia
- Pneumonia

Your medical team will monitor you in order to minimize these risks, and provide instructions for ways you can minimize risk of complications as well.

Future trends in surgery

Healthcare is proving to be one of the promising areas in which new AR and virtual reality technologies can be used to change long-established surgical procedures. It's like using a kind of GPS with augmented reality to navigate to a specific point in the human body.

The Real-Time, Fused Holographic Visualization system that puts a Microsoft HoloLens onto the face of the lead surgeon is like a missile-guidance system. It lets the surgeon plan out a digital path to the patient's tumor, which also improves patient experience and understanding of what will be done during their procedure. During surgery, like in a comic book or on Star Trek, a surgeon wearing the HoloLens can look directly at their patient and see all of the patient's internal anatomy under their skin.

Liver transplantation

Liver transplantation, replacing the diseased liver with a cadaveric or a living donor liver, plays an increasing role in treatment of hepato cellular carcinoma. Although outcomes following liver transplant were initially poor (20%–36% survival rate), outcomes have significantly improved with improvement in surgical techniques and adoption of the Milan criteria at US transplantation centers.

The risks of liver transplantation extend beyond risk of the procedure itself. The immunosuppressive medication required after surgery to prevent rejection of the donor liver also impairs the body's natural ability to combat dysfunctional cells. If the tumor has spread undetected outside the liver before the transplant, the medication effectively increases the rate of disease progression and decreases survival. With this in mind, liver transplant "can be a curative approach for patients with advanced HCC without extrahepatic metastasis". Patient selection is considered a major key for success.

The potential side effects of immune-suppressing drugs include:

- High blood pressure
- High cholesterol
- Kidney problems
- Diabetes
- Bone weakening (called osteoporosis)

Ablation

Radiofrequency ablation (RFA)

RFA uses high-frequency radio waves to destroy tumor by local heating. The electrodes are inserted into the liver tumor under ultrasound image guidance using percutaneous, laparoscopic or open surgical approach. It is suitable for small tumors

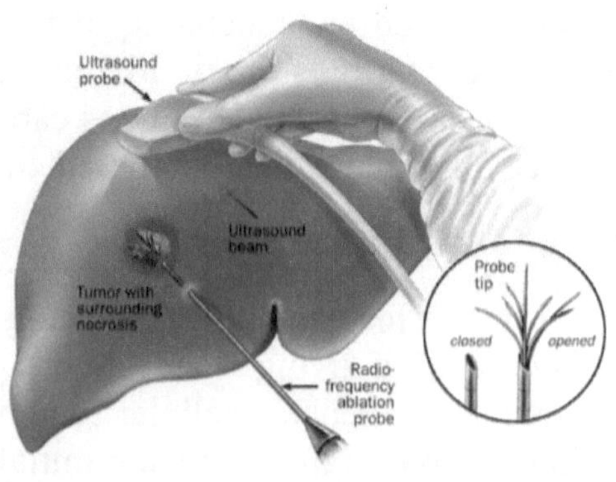

(<5 cm). RFA has the best outcomes in patients with a solitary tumor less than 4 cm. Since it is a local treatment and has minimal effect on normal healthy tissue, it can be repeated multiple times. Survival is better for those with smaller tumors. In one study, In one series of 302 patients, the three-year survival rates for lesions >5 cm, 2.1 to 5 cm, and ≤2 cm were 59, 74, and 91%, respectively. A large randomized trial comparing surgical resection and RFA for small HCC showed similar four-year survival and less morbidities for patients treated with RFA.

Cryoablation

This is a technique used to destroy tissue using cold temperature. The tumor is not removed and the destroyed cancer is left to be reabsorbed by the body. Initial results in properly selected patients with unresectable liver tumors are equivalent to those of resection. Cryosurgery involves the placement of a stainless steel probe into the center of the tumor. Liquid nitrogen is circulated through the end of this device. The tumor and a half inch margin of normal liver are frozen to −190 °C for 15 minutes, which is lethal to all tissues. The area is thawed for 10 minutes and then refrozen to −190°C for another 15 minutes. After the tumor has thawed, the probe is removed, bleeding is controlled, and the procedure is complete. The patient spends the first postoperative night in the intensive care unit and typically is discharged in 3–5 days. Proper selection of patients and attention to detail in performing the cryosurgical procedure are mandatory to achieve good results and outcomes. Frequently, cryosurgery is used in conjunction with liver resection, as some of the tumors are removed while others are treated with cryosurgery.

Percutaneous ethanol injection is well tolerated, with high RR in small (<3 cm) solitary tumors

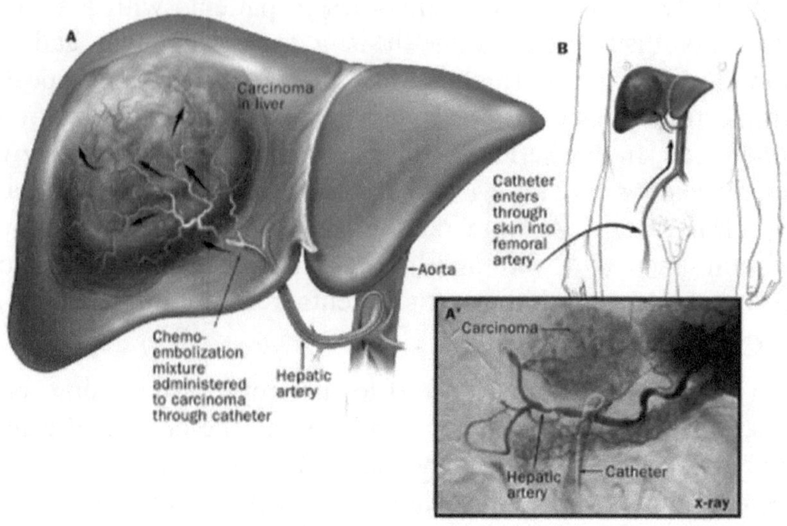

Arterial catheter-based treatment

Transcatheter arterial chemoembolization (TACE) This performed for unresectable tumors or as a temporary treatment while waiting for liver transplant ("bridge to transplant"). TACE is done by injecting an antineoplastic drug (e.g. cisplatin) mixed with a radio-opaque contrast (e.g. Lipiodol) and an embolic agent (e.g. Gelfoam) into the right or left hepatic artery via the groin artery. The goal of the procedure is to restrict the tumor's vascular supply while supplying a targeted chemotherapeutic agent. TACE has been shown to increase survival and to downstage HCC in patients who exceed the Milan criteria for liver transplant. Patients who undergo the procedure are followed with CT scans and may need additional TACE procedures if the tumor persists. As of 2005, multiple trials show objective tumor responses and slowed tumor progression, but questionable survival benefit compared to supportive care; greatest benefit is seen in people with preserved liver function, absence of vascular invasion, and smallest tumors. TACE is not suitable for big tumors (>8 cm), the presence of portal vein thrombus, tumors with a portal-systemic shunt, and patients with poor liver function.

Selective internal radiation therapy (SIRT) can be used to destroy the tumor from within (thus minimizing exposure to healthy tissue). Similar to TACE, this is a procedure in which an interventional radiologist selectively injects the artery or arteries supplying the tumor with a chemotherapeutic agent. The agent is typically Yttrium-90 (Y-90) incorporated into embolic microspheres that lodge in the tumor vasculature, causing ischemia and delivering their radiation dose directly to the lesion. This technique allows for a higher, local dose of radiation to be delivered directly to the tumor while sparing normal healthy tissue. While not curative, patients have increased survival. No studies have been done to compare whether SIRT is superior to TACE in terms of survival outcomes, although retrospective studies suggest similar efficacy. Two products are available, SIR-Spheres and TheraSphere. The latter is an FDA approved treatment for primary liver cancer (HCC) which has been shown in clinical trials to increase the survival rate of low-risk patients. SIR-Spheres are FDA approved for the treatment of metastatic colorectal cancer, but outside the US, SIR-Spheres are approved for the treatment of any nonresectable liver cancer including primary liver cancer.

Chemotherapy

Systemic chemotherapy remains the mainstay of therapy for patients with advanced HCC who are not candidates for surgical resection, liver transplantation, or localized tumor ablation. Unfortunately, HCC is minimally responsive to systemic chemotherapy. Resistance to chemotherapy may be caused by the universal expression of the multidrug resistance gene protein on the surface of the malignant cells, leading to active efflux of chemotherapeutic agents.

Chemotherapy is usually not well tolerated and seems to be less efficacious in patients with HCC who have underlying hepatic dysfunction. Younger patients with well-compensated cirrhosis due to chronic hepatitis B or C infections have better outcomes with chemotherapy than older patients with alcoholic cirrhosis and other comorbid diseases.

The most active drugs tested for single-agent therapy have been doxorubicin, cisplatin, and fluorouracil. Response rates are about 10%, and treatment shows no clear impact on overall survival. The combination of gemcitabine and oxaliplatin (GEMOX) helped to shrink large hepatomas to the point where some could be resected, according to a multicenter retrospective study in France.

There is also no apparent benefit to chemotherapy in the adjuvant setting following resection or radiofrequency ablation (RFA). In an effort to provide care in this difficult population, various hormonal and biologic agents have been tried with minimal success, including tamoxifen, antiandrogens (e.g., cyproterone and ketoconazole), interferon, interleukin (IL)-2, and octreotide. Currently, liver-directed therapies (e.g., resection, transplantation, and RFA) offer the only genuine hope for extended survival in patients with advanced HCC.

Sorafenib

Sorafenib is an oral agent that has antiangiogenic, proapoptotic, and Raf-kinase inhibitory properties. In 2007, it was approved by the US Food and Drug Administration (FDA) for use in patients with unresectable HCC. Sorafenib is regarded as a standard medical treatment for advanced HCC. In addition, data from the TACTICS trial suggest that adding it to TACE may lead to improved survival as compared with TACE alone in patients with unresectable HCC.

For people who cannot tolerate sorafenib, or as an alternative first-line therapy, a similar drug called Lenvima (lenvatinib) may be considered.

In a phase III study, Lenvima (when compared to sorafenib) had a higher overall survival benefit (13.6 months versus 12.3), higher response rate (24 percent versus 9 percent), and a higher time to disease progression (7.4 months versus 3.7 months).

The most common side effects of Lenvima are:

- High blood pressure
- Diarrhea
- Decreased appetite
- Weight loss
- Fatigue

Another targeted drug Stivarga (regorafenib) blocks proteins that help liver cancer cells grow. This drug is currently used as a second-line therapy (meaning if sorafenib or Lenvima stop working).

Common side effects include:

- Fatigue
- Loss of appetite and weight loss
- Rash on hands and feet
- High blood pressure
- Fever and infections
- Diarrhea
- Belly pain

Other drugs

The following additional systemic drug options exist for patients with HCC who have stopped responding to initial treatment with sorafenib, Lenvatinib or Regorafenib:

- Nivolumab
- Pembrolizumab

- Cabozantinib
- Ramucirumab

Other Procedures

Portal vein embolization (PVE): This technique is sometimes used to increase the volume of healthy liver, in order to improve chances of survival following surgical removal of diseased liver. For example, embolization of the right main portal vein would result in compensatory hypertrophy of the left lobe, which may qualify the patient for a partial hepatectomy. Embolization is performed by an interventional radiologist using a percutaneous transhepatic approach. This procedure can also serve as a bridge to transplant.

High intensity focused ultrasound (HIFU) (as opposed to diagnostic ultrasound) is an experimental technique which uses high-powered ultrasound waves to destroy tumor tissue.

A systematic review assessed 12 articles involving a total of 318 patients with hepatocellular carcinoma treated with Yttrium-90 radioembolization. Excluding a study of only one patient, post-treatment CT evaluation of the tumor showed a response ranging from 29 to 100% of patients evaluated, with all but two studies showing a response of 71% or greater.

Treatment of Complications

Jaundice

Treatment of jaundice is based on the cause of the elevated bilirubin level. When jaundice is caused by a tumor or cirrhosis, treatment may include:

- Surgery to remove the obstruction
- Placing a thin plastic or metal tube (called a stent) to allow the bile to drain around the obstruction

- Jaundice can cause itching. You can try applying unscented and hypoallergenic skin lotions and lubricants several times a day to relieve itching.
- Anti-itching medicines like antihistamines. In some cases, an antidepressant may help

Portal Hypertension

Treatment of portal hypertension is aimed at prevention of complications. The main goal of therapy is to decrease portal pressure. This is generally difficult to achieve and adequately maintain.

Ascites is the presence of excess fluid in the peritoneal cavity.

- Fluid restriction to less than 1.5 liters per day
- Diuretic therapy - combination of spironolactone with a loop diuretic (Lasix)
- Abdominal Paracentesis in which a needle is inserted into the peritoneal cavity and ascitic fluid is removed

Esophageal Varices are swolen veins that occur in the esophagus or stomach as a result of portal hypertension. Varices often rupture and bleed profusely and cause hemetemesis (vomiting of blood) and 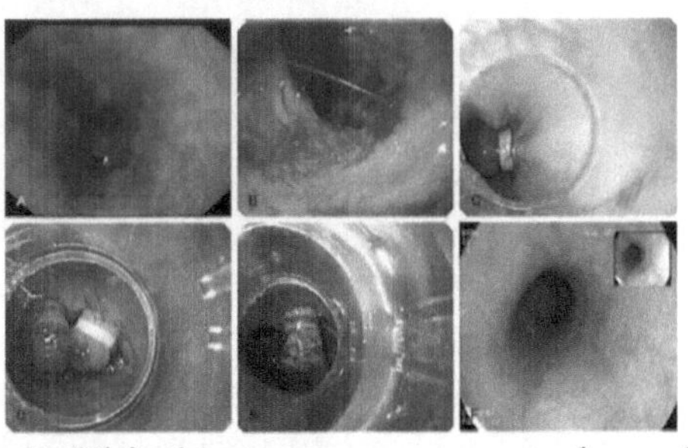 melena (dark black, tarry feces). This is an emergency and need immediate treatment in a well equipped center.

- **Betablocker** – Propranolol
- **Vasopressin** in the acutely bleeding patient is effective and works by decreasing splanchnic blood flow. Vasopressin therapy should be instituted in an intensive

care unit through a central venous access line. Vasopressin should be administered with sublingual nitroglycerin. Somatostatin is currently the preferred drug for acute variceal bleeding.

- **Antibiotics**
- **Blood transfusion**
- **Endoscopic Therapy**
  - o **Banding** - Acute variceal hemorrhage is ideally managed by variceal ligation with elastic rings, commonly called banding.

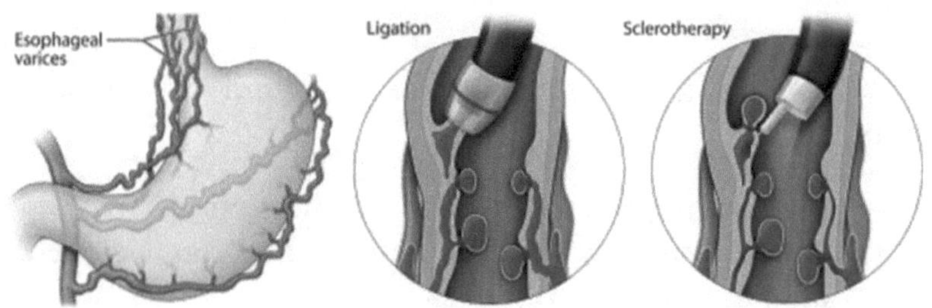

  - o **Sclerotherapy** - The use of sclerotherapy, or injection of a sclerosing agent directly into and around the varices, has been well studied. The technique consists of injecting 1–10 mL of sclerosing agent (sodium morrhuate, sodium tetradecyl sulfate, ethanolamine oleate, or absolute alcohol) into the varix beginning at the gastroesophageal junction and circumferentially into all columns.
  - o **Balloon Tamponade** - Balloon tamponade is useful to control variceal bleeding through compression. Use of one of three commercially available balloons to tamponade bleeding esophageal or gastric varices can be employed when medical management has not been successful, and endoscopic management has failed or is unavailable.
  - o **Shunting Procedures** - Nonsurgical Transjugular Intrahepatic Portal-Systemic Shunt (TIPSS) This is a

radiologic procedure that has become very popular as an alternative method of controlling acute bleeding, especially if gastric varices are present. It is also indicated in patients who have had recurrent bleeding despite medical or endoscopic management. Contraindications to TIPSS placement include severe liver dysfunction, renal failure, and heart failure.

o Surgical Shunts -The aim of surgical shunting in portal hypertension is threefold: 1) to reduce portal venous pressure, 2) to maintain hepatic and portal blood flow, and 3) to try to reduce or not complicate hepatic encephalopathy. Currently, there is no procedure that reliably and consistently fulfills all of these criteria.

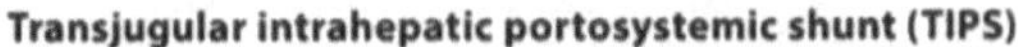

Transjugular intrahepatic portosystemic shunt (TIPS)

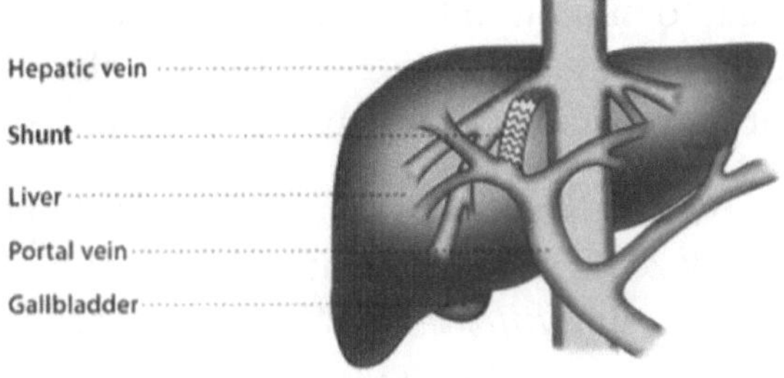

Hepatic Encephalopathy

Hepatic encephalopathy is a decline in brain function that occurs as a result of severe liver disease. In this condition, your liver can't adequately remove toxins from your blood. This causes a buildup of toxins in your bloodstream, which can lead to brain damage.

- Exclude nonhepatic causes of altered mental function.

- Consider checking an *arterial ammonia level* in the initial assessment of a hospitalized patient and precipitants of hepatic encephalopathy, such as hypovolemia, metabolic disturbances, gastrointestinal bleeding, infection, and constipation, should be corrected.

- Avoid medications that depress central nervous system function, especially *benzodiazepines*. Patients with severe agitation and hepatic encephalopathy may receive *haloperidol* as a sedative

- Patients with severe encephalopathy who are at risk for aspiration should undergo prophylactic endotracheal intubation.

- **Lactulose** 30 mL twice daily or more may be administered orally or by nasogastric tube. Lactulose appears to inhibit intestinal ammonia production by a number of mechanisms. Lactulose also works as a cathartic, reducing colonic bacterial load.

- **Antibiotics** - Neomycin and other antibiotics, such as metronidazole, oral vancomycin, paromomycin, oral quinolones, and *Rifaximin* are administered in an effort to decrease the colonic concentration of ammoniagenic bacteria. Initial neomycin dosing is 250 mg orally 2-4 times a day. Doses as high as 4000 mg/d may be administered.

- **L-ornithine L-aspartate** (LOLA) (Hepa-Merz) as both orally or intravenously.

- **Sodium phenylbutyrate** (Buphenyl), intravenous sodium phenylacetate in combination with sodium benzoate (Ammonul), and glycerol phenylbutyrate (Ravicti).

- **L-carnitine and zinc.**

Prognosis

Overall prognosis for survival is poor, with a 5-year relative survival rate of 18%. In patients diagnosed with a localized stage of disease, the 5-year survival is 31%. Length of survival depends largely on the extent of cirrhosis in the liver; cirrhotic patients have shorter survival times and more limited therapeutic options. Portal vein occlusion, which occurs commonly, portends an even shorter survival.

The influence of diabetes, obesity, and glycemic control continues to be evaluated in studies of the etiology and outcomes of HCC. For example, in a study of patients who had undergone curative resection for solitary HCV-related HCC, the tumor-free survival rate at 3 years was more than twice as high in patients in patients who had a normal hemoglobin A1c than in those whose hemoglobin A1c was 6.5% or higher (66% versus 27%).

Complications from HCC are those of hepatic failure; death occurs from cachexia, variceal bleeding, or (rarely) tumor rupture and bleeding into the peritoneum. Signs and symptoms of hepatic failure may signify tumor recurrence and/or progression.

Various studies have reported extrahepatic metastasis in up to 30–50% of cases of HCC, with lungs the commonest site, followed by lymph nodes and bones. Unusual extrahepatic metastatic sites include the following:

- Adrenal glands
- Peritoneum
- Diaphragm
- Soft tissues
- Brain
- Skin
- Oral cavity

Prevention

While it's not always possible to prevent liver cancer, you can reduce your risk by being vaccinated against hepatitis B, being tested for hepatitis C, practicing safe sex, and limiting your consumption of alcohol. Other measures may reduce your risk even further.

Together, hepatitis B and hepatitis C infections are responsible for 85 percent to 90 percent of liver cancers, so taking measures to prevent these infections, and seeking treatment for them if present, is a great way to not only reduce your risk of liver cancer but other related diseases.

Vaccination

Unfortunately, there is no vaccine for hepatitis C. The hepatitis B vaccine, however, is recommended for all children in the United States and is required by schools for admission.

If you are a young adult, review your medical records to ensure you were properly immunized as a child. If you don't have those records, speak with your doctor about whether getting the hepatitis B vaccination is right for you. Other adults who have not been immunized may want to consider being vaccinated as well, especially if they have any risk factors for acquiring the disease.

It's currently recommended that all healthcare professionals receive the vaccine, as well as anyone else who may have contact with blood.

Risk factors for hepatitis B include having multiple sex partners, using injectable (illicit) drugs, having a sexually transmitted disease (including HIV), having a chronic liver disease, and having diabetes under the age of 60. Given rates of hepatitis B outside of the United States, adults who were born overseas are also at risk as the virus can be transferred from mother to baby during childbirth or breastfeeding, often resulting in a chronic infection.

What many people do not realize is that it is relatively easy to contract the hepatitis B virus, unlike viruses such as HIV.

Simply sharing a toothbrush or having small cuts on your hand and touching a doorknob with a trace amount of blood from someone with hepatitis B is enough to contract the infection.

Roughly 95 percent of people who become infected with the hepatitis B virus clear the virus, though they may become very ill. The other 5 percent become chronic carriers of the disease. They are often not ill when they acquired it and may otherwise be unaware of the infection until it does substantial damage (including that which leads to liver cancer).

Testing

Testing for diseases that can lead to liver cancer can go a long way in catching these risk factors early in an attempt to prevent them from progressing in this way.

Hepatitis B and C Testing

If you were born between 1945 and 1965, have your blood tested for hepatitis C. Other people who have risk factors, such as those discussed for hepatitis B, should be tested as well.

Hepatitis C is the leading cause of liver cancer in the United States, Europe, and Japan.

People who are infected with hepatitis C are much more likely to become carriers than those infected with hepatitis B, and 10 percent to 30 percent of people who contract the infection will go on to develop cirrhosis.

The hepatitis C virus was only discovered in 1989, and testing of blood used for transfusions for hepatitis C has only been done since the 1990s. What this means, is that anyone who had a blood transfusion prior to that time could be at risk, hence the testing recommendations.

If it is determined that a person carries hepatitis C, medications are available that can clear the virus in up to 99 percent of people.

This means that even if you are positive, you may be able to prevent cirrhosis and reduce your risk of liver cancer.

If it's determined that someone is a carrier of hepatitis B, there are medications that can reduce the risk of developing cirrhosis (and likely liver cancer) as well.

But in order to be treated, you need to know you carry the virus.

Hemochromatosis Testing

Having a family member who has or had liver cancer increases your risk, but so does having a number of different genetic diseases, some that you may not be aware you carry. Hemochromatosis—excessive absorption and storage of iron that leads to cirrhosis and, in time, liver cancer—is one of them.

If you have a family history of people who had liver disease (not just liver cancer) but who were not big drinkers of alcohol, talk to your doctor about being tested for the disease. Other family members may thank you as well, as the condition is currently greatly underdiagnosed.

There are other genetic diseases, though much less common, that raise the risk of liver cancer. It's important to know your genetic blueprint so that your doctor can properly test you for others that may be related to liver cancer or other health conditions.

Safe Sex

Both hepatitis B and hepatitis C can be passed sexually. The consistent use of condoms can greatly reduce your risk of contracting not only hepatitis but other sexually transmitted infections, including HIV.

If you have hepatitis B, you should advise your partner so that he or she can get vaccinated. Even after vaccination, condoms should still be used. Your partner can be tested to see if he or she is immune six months after the final dose.

If you don't have hepatitis B, you can further reduce your risk by cutting down on your number of sex partners.

If you have hepatitis C, you should use condoms. If you are treated, and eventually clear the virus, you may be able to stop (though this is only advised if you are in a monogamous relationship). Hepatitis C is less likely to be transmitted sexually than hepatitis B, but it is still possible.

Reduced Alcohol Intake

Drinking excessive amounts of alcohol can cause the progressive scarring of liver tissue, a condition known as cirrhosis. If drinking continues, the condition can progress from compensated cirrhosis (meaning the liver can still function to some degree) to decompensated cirrhosis (where the liver no longer works).

The bottom line is this: Cirrhosis greatly increases your risk of liver failure, and long-term heavy alcohol use (more than three drinks daily) can increase your risk of liver cancer as well.

Smoking Cessation

If you are a smoker, now is the time to quit. In addition to increasing your risk of heart disease, stroke, and other cancers, smoking can increase your risk of liver cancer.

A 2018 study found that while smoking increased the risk of liver cancer by around 25 percent, the combination of smoking plus being a carrier of the hepatitis B virus was much more than additive in terms of your risk increase.

Those who were carriers of hepatitis B but had never smoked were 7.6 times more likely to develop liver cancer, whereas for those who had hepatitis B and had ever smoked, the risk was 15.68 times greater than average.

Careful Needle Use

A large number of hepatitis C infections (as well as many hepatitis B infections) are caused by injection drug use (IDU). With no vaccine to protect against hepatitis C (or HIV), the only sure way to avoid IDU infection is to either not inject drugs or to avoid sharing needles and syringes. This includes the shared use of drug paraphernalia, such as cotton, spoons, and other cooking instruments.

If you choose to continue injecting drugs, you should access free needle exchange programs offered by many state and municipal public health authorities. Consider, though, that injection drug use not only increases your risk of getting hepatitis but may speed up liver disease progression—meaning that your risk of liver cirrhosis and cancer is all the more profound.

The problem of liver cancer related to IDU is not going away. Another 2018 study found that between 1990 and 2016, the global number of liver cancers attributable to injection drug use rose more than threefold.

Shared tattoo needles are also a potential source of infection (with both the hepatitis viruses and HIV).

If you get a tattoo, make sure the tattoo artist uses new needles. While it's law in the United States that new needles must be used, it's wise to check just in case.

Water Checks

Well water can be a source of *arsenic*, a carcinogen known to cause liver cancer. Arsenic can also cause kidney damage, heart disease, and problems with brain development in children. It can enter groundwater through natural processes in the environment, but also as a contaminant from pesticides and industrial waste.

Arsenic in untreated well water has been found in all regions of the United States.

Certainly arsenic in well water is low on the list of potential causes of liver cancer, but, in addition to other problems related to arsenic, there are other reasons you should test your well water. Additional contaminants can include other heavy metals, organic chemicals, nitrates and nitrites, and microorganisms, which can contribute to other health concerns.

Workplace Safety

Some individuals are at increased risk of being exposed to chemicals associated with liver cancer due to the nature of their work or workplace.

Chemicals of concern with regard to liver cancer include:

- Acrylamide
- Benzo(a)pyrene (BaP)
- Dichlorodiphenyltrichloroethane (DDT)
- Perchlorethylene
- Perfluorinated chemicals (PFCs)
- Perfluorooctanoic acid (PFOA)
- Polychlorinated biphenyls (PCBs)
- Trichloroethylene
- Vinyl chloride (causes angiosarcoma of the liver)

Some of the lines of work that may involve these exposures include:

- Aerospace
- Construction/home repair (cabling, house framing, plumbing)
- Dry cleaning
- Farming
- Food packaging
- Gasoline
- Manufacturing (plastics, chemicals, and rubber; e.g. electronics, pharmaceuticals, shoes)

- Metal working
- Motor vehicle repair
- Printing
- PVC fabrication
- Textile processing

Employers are required to provide Material Safety Data Sheets (MSDSs) on any chemicals you may be exposed to at the workplace. It's important to read and follow any precautions, such as the use of gloves, a respirator, and more. The National Institute for Occupational Safety and Health has a very handy pocket guide to chemical hazards that can provide more information.

If you have concerns about your workplace, you can contact the National Institute for Occupational Safety and Health (OSHA).

Weight Reduction

Obesity (or being overweight) hasn't been directly linked to liver cancer, but it is a risk factor for a few conditions that are, in turn, risk factors for liver cancer themselves.

Non-alcoholic fatty liver disease is a condition often associated with obesity. The condition is associated with a four-fold increased risk of developing liver cancer.

Type 2 diabetes is also a risk factor for liver cancer. Since type 2 diabetes is strongly associated with being overweight, this is yet another reason to watch your weight.

People who have type 2 diabetes have three times the likelihood of developing liver cancer.

If losing weight sounds daunting, keep in mind that losing even five to 10 pounds has been found to make a difference when it comes to many health conditions. Losing 7 percent of body weight improves the way your body uses insulin and reduces insulin resistance.

Rather than just reducing the amount of food you eat (while that is important), take a moment to learn about what it takes to takes to lose weight and keep it off to raise your chances of being successful.

Alternative cancer treatments

We are fighting with cancer since the dawn of history. Every year we discover new diagnostic modalities, better radiotherapy techniques and lots of new chemotherapy drugs. But we have completely failed to defeat this disease called cancer. Think again, are we really going on the right path? Does conventional Medicine really targets upon the prime cause of cancer?

It's not that more effective alternative treatments for cancer don't exist – they most certainly do. It's just that the allopathic system isn't at all interested in divulging real cures. This is because their expensive therapies generate billions of dollars for the cancer industry.

Chemotherapy Doesn't Cure Cancer – It Causes It!

Chemotherapy does, in fact, kill cancer cells. But it also kills healthy cells, along with a patient's immune system and, really, anything else that crosses its path. At worst, such treatments kill patients more quickly than if they had chosen not to undergo them at all.

There's no money to be made in prescribing prevention advice like eating fewer chemicals and exercising more. The "bread and butter" of the cancer industry is unleashing the next, latest-and-greatest cancer drug. Not telling you how to avoid cancer in the first place.

Many people with cancer are interested in trying any treatment that may cure them safely, including complementary and alternative cancer treatments. There is growing evidence that these alternative cancer treatments give wonderful results. Here are some alternative cancer treatments that are very safe and effective.

- **Budwig Protocol -** *The best Alternative Treatment effective in all cancers and all stages with documented 90% success*
- Laetrile (Vitamin B-17) Therapy
- Gerson Therapy
- Dr. Simoncini Baking Soda Cancer Treatment
- High-dose vitamin C
- Frankincense Essential Oil Therapy
- Immunotherapy
- Hyperthermia
- Oxygen Therapy and Hyperbaric Chambers

Laetrile (Vitamin B-17) Therapy

Introduction

During 1950, after many years of research, a dedicated biochemist Dr. Ernest T. Krebs Jr., isolated a new vitamin from bitter apricot kernel that he called 'B-17' or 'Laetrile'. He conducted further lab animal and culture experiments to conclude that laetrile would be effective in the treatment of cancer. As the years rolled by, thousands became convinced that Krebs had finally found the treatment for all cancers. He proposed that cancer was caused by a deficiency of Vitamin B 17 (Laetrile, Amygdaline).

To prove that it was not toxic to humans he injected it into his own arm. As he predicted, there were no harmful or distressing side effects. The Laetrile had no harmful effect on normal cells but was deadly to cancer cells. Dr. Ernst Krebs stated that we need at least a minimum of 100 mg of B-17 or around 7 bitter apricot seeds to almost guarantee a cancer free life.

Nitriloside is a beta-cyanophoric glycosides, a large group of water-soluble, sugar-containing compounds found in a number of plants. Amygdalin is one of the most common nitrilosides. Laetrile is a partly man-made molecule and shares only part of the Amygdalin structure. Both Laetrile and Amygdalin have been promoted as "Vitamin B-17".

Laetrile stands for laevo-rotatory mandelonitrile beta-diglucoside. The "laevo" part references a purified form of B-17 that turns polarized light in a left-turning direction. Dr. Krebs, Jr. believed that only the left-rotating Laevo form was effective against cancer. So it's important to check the purity of your Laetrile.

How B-17 works (A tale of two enzymes)

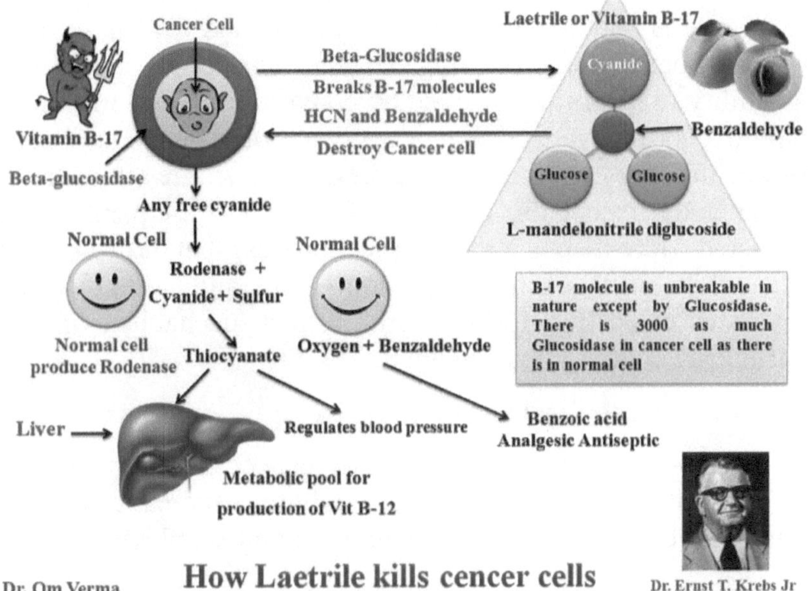

Laetrile, commonly known as Vitamin B-17 or Amygdalin, contains two units of Sugar, one of Benzaldehyde and one of Cyanide, all tightly locked within it. Everyone knows that cyanide can be highly toxic and even fatal if taken in sufficient quantity. However, as it is in locked state is completely inert and absolutely has no effect on living tissue. There is only one substance that can unlock this molecule and release the cyanide. That substance is an enzyme called beta-glucocidase, which we shall call the unlocking enzyme. When B-17 comes in contact with this enzyme, not only the cyanide is released but also Benzaldehyde which is highly toxic by itself. In fact, these two working together are at least 100 times more poisonous to cancer cell than either of them separately. The unlocking enzyme is not found to any dangerous degree anywhere in the body except at

79

the cancer cell where it is present in great quantity. The result is that Vit B-17 is unlocked at the cancer cells becomes poisonous to the cancer cells and only to the cancer cells.

There is another important enzyme called Rodanese, which we shall identify as protecting enzyme. The reason is that it has the ability to neutralize cyanide by converting it instantly into the byproducts (thiocyanate) that actually are beneficial and essential for health. This enzyme is found in great quantities in every part of the body except the cancer cells which consequently is not protected. Here then is a biochemical process that destroys cancer cells while at the same time nourishing and sustaining non-cancerous cells. It is intricate and perfect mechanism of nature that simply couldn't be accidental.

Laetrile - Metabolic Therapy

Metabolic therapy is a non-toxic cancer treatment based on the use of Vitamin B- 17, proteolytic pancreatic enzymes, immuno-stimulants, and vitamin and mineral supplements.

There are three parts to this program:
1. Laetrile
2. Vitamins and enzymes
3. Diet

Phase I Metabolic - Program for the first 21 days

Laetrile

Amygdalin (Laetrile) is available in 500 mg. tablets and in vials (10 cc 3 Gm) for intravenous use. Both forms are used. Two vials of Laetrile are given IV three times weekly for three weeks with at least one day between injections (Mon., Wed., Fri.). Dose of Amygdalin Tablets 500 mg is 2 tab three times a day with meals on the days on which the patients do not receive the intravenous Laetrile. Thiocyanate levels in the blood can be measured during treatment. In general, the patients who do best are those in whom the thiocyanate level is between 1.2 and 2.5 Mg/DL (Philip E.Binzel   ).

Vitamins and Enzymes

Preven-Ca Caps - Preven-Ca is a comprehensive blend of potent herb and fruit extracts, designed to provide a broad Spectrum of Flavonoids with scientifically demonstrated Antioxidant activity and effectiveness. One capsule with each meal.

Vitamin B15 - One capsule three times a daily at the end of each meal.

Megazyme Forte (Proteolytic Enzymes) Three tablets two hours after each meal (9 daily).

Ester Vitamin C 1000 mg capsule - One capsule with each meal.

Shark Cartilage It has been said that Sharks are the healthiest creature on earth. Sharks are immune to practically every disease known to man. One capsules three times a daily with each meal.

Natural Vitamin E 400 iu - One gel with lunch and one with dinner.

AHCC (Active Hexose Correlated Compound) - Two capsules with each meal.

Multi Vitamin & Mineral Liquid - 1 oz (two tablespoons) once daily with a meal.

Vitamin A & E Emulsion - 5 drops in juice or water three times per day.

Barley Grass Juice - One teaspoon in juice three times per day.

Bitter apricot seeds - No more than 12 every 2 hours 6 times a day.

Dimethyl sulfoxide (DMSO) - DMSO is a by-product of the wood and paper industry. It is known for its ability to permeate living tissue and stimulate cellular processes.

Or Phase 1 Oral

Injectable Amygdalin is replaced with 500mg Amygdalin tablets. Binzel recommends 2 of these tablets with each meal for a total of 6 per day. Otherwise the ORAL Phase 1 includes the same materials as above.

Phase 2 Metabolic - Program for the next 3 months

It comprises the same materials as Phase 1 except that the dosages for the vitamin B-17 as well as the A&E Emulsion Drops change to the following:

Vitamin B-17 500 mg tablets: 1 tablet with each meal and one at bedtime.

Vitamin A & E emulsion drops: 10 drops in juice or water two times per day (suspend for 2 months after 3 months of use).

Diet

Consume those fruits (i.e. seeds), grains and nuts that are rich in laetrile. Consume salads with healthy dressings. For protein patient should consume whole grains including corn, beans, buckwheat, nuts, dried fruits. Real butter in small amounts is permitted. The patients are not permitted anything which contains white flour or white sugar. Take away all meat, all poultry, all fish, all eggs and milk from patients. Margarine is detrimental to good nutrition. No coffee is permitted.

Zinc acts as transport vehicle for laetrile in the body. If patient does not have sufficient zinc, laetrile will not get into the tissues of the body. That's why you should give a spoonful of pumpkin seeds along with bitter apricot kernels. The body will not rebuild any tissue without sufficient quantities of Vitamin C etc.

The Gerson Therapy

The Gerson Therapy is a natural treatment that activates the body's extraordinary ability to heal itself through an organic, plant-based diet, raw juices, coffee enemas and natural supplements.

With its whole-body approach to healing, the Gerson Therapy naturally reactivates your body's magnificent ability to heal itself – with no damaging side effects. This a powerful, natural treatment boosts the body's own immune system to heal cancer, arthritis, heart disease, allergies, and many other degenerative diseases. Dr. Max Gerson developed the Gerson Therapy in the 1930s, initially as a treatment for his own debilitating migraines, and eventually as a treatment for degenerative diseases such as skin tuberculosis, diabetes and, most famously, cancer.

An abundance of nutrients from copious amounts of fresh, organic juices are consumed every day, providing your body with a super-dose of enzymes, minerals and nutrients. These substances then break down diseased tissue in the body, while coffee enemas aid in eliminating toxins from the liver.

Throughout our lives our bodies are being filled with a variety of carcinogens and toxic pollutants. These toxins reach us through the air we breathe, the food we eat, the medicines we take and the water we drink. The Gerson Therapy's intensive detoxification regimen eliminates these toxins from the body, so that true healing can begin.

How the Gerson Therapy Works

The Gerson Therapy regenerates the body to health, supporting each important metabolic requirement by flooding the body with nutrients from about 15- 20 pounds of organically-grown fruits and vegetables daily. Most is used to make fresh raw juice, up to one glass every hour, up to 13 times per day. Raw and cooked solid foods are generously consumed. Oxygenation is usually more than doubled, as oxygen deficiency in the blood contributes to many degenerative diseases. The metabolism is also stimulated through the addition of thyroid, potassium and other supplements, and by avoiding heavy animal fats, excess protein, sodium and other toxins.

Degenerative diseases render the body increasingly unable to excrete waste materials adequately, commonly resulting in liver and kidney failure. The Gerson Therapy uses intensive detoxification to eliminate wastes, regenerate the liver, reactivate the immune system and restore the body's essential defenses – enzyme, mineral and hormone systems. With generous, high-quality nutrition, increased oxygen availability, detoxification, and improved metabolism, the cells – and the body – can regenerate, become healthy and prevent future illness.

Juicing

Fresh-pressed juice from raw foods provides the easiest and most effective way of providing high-quality nutrition. By juicing, patients can take in the nutrients and enzymes from nearly 15 pounds of produce every day, in a manner that is easy to digest and absorb.

Every day, a typical patient on the Gerson Therapy for cancer consumes up to thirteen glasses of fresh, raw carrot-apple and green leaf juices. These juices are prepared hourly from fresh, raw, organic fruits and vegetables, using a two-step juicer or a masticating juicer used with a separate hydraulic press.

The Gerson Therapy Diet

The Gerson Therapy diet is plant-based and entirely organic. The diet is naturally high in vitamins, minerals, enzymes, micro-nutrients, and extremely low in sodium, fats, and proteins. The following is a typical daily diet for a Gerson patient on the full therapy regimen:

- Thirteen glasses of fresh, raw carrot-apple and green-leaf juices prepared hourly from fresh, organic fruits and vegetables.
- Three full plant-based meals, freshly prepared from organically grown fruits, vegetables and whole grains. A typical meal will include salad, cooked vegetables, baked potatoes, Hippocrates soup and juice.
- Fresh fruit and vegetables available at all hours for snacking, in addition to the regular diet.

Supplements

All medications used in connection with the Gerson Therapy are classed as biologicals, materials of organic origin that are supplied in therapeutic amounts. The supplements used on the Gerson Therapy include:

- Potassium compound
- Lugol's solution
- Vitamin B-12
- Thyroid hormone
- Pancreatic Enzymes

Detoxification

Coffee enemas are the primary method of detoxification of the tissues and blood on the Gerson Therapy. Coffee enemas accomplish this essential task, assisting the liver in eliminating toxic residues from the body for good. Cancer patients on the Gerson Therapy may take up to 5 coffee enemas per day. The Gerson Therapy also utilizes castor oil to stimulate bile flow and enhance the liver's ability to filter blood.

Simoncini's Baking Soda Cancer Treatment

Dr. Tullio Simoncini is a medical doctor in Italy who has done more than anyone to explore the uses of the baking soda cancer treatment as an alternative cancer treatment. It is known that cancer creates and favors an acid environment and because of this, Dr. Simoncini and others have used sodium bicarbonate as an alkaline therapeutic agent.

The way that acidity seems to protect cancer is not fully understood. It seems that cytotoxic T-cells, which may attack cancer cells under normal conditions, are inactivated in an acid extracellular fluid. Also, the type of acidity that cancer produces, i.e., lactic acid, stimulates vascular endothelial growth factor and angiogenesis. This is like a highway project, which enables a tumor to build the blood vessels that it needs to bring the nutrients for it to survive. So the tumor creates an environment in which it can then exist comfortably.

Baking Soda's Alkalinity Fights Cancer's Acidity

At a pH of about 10, sodium bicarbonate is an antidote to this acidity. It can be used clinically in sterile, intravenous form. This is a liquid, sterile bicarbonate of soda. The baking soda cancer treatment is well-tolerated, even with frequent repeated dosing. Dr. Simonchini also injects soda bicarb solution directly into the tumors at his center.

Cancer a Fungus problem?

Dr. Simonchini says that cancer is caused by fungus However, it is useful to know that not only does sodium bicarbonate disrupt the comfortable environment of tumors, but it also has anti-fungal effect.

Best Alternative Treatment - Budwig Protocol

90% documented success in all types of Cancers

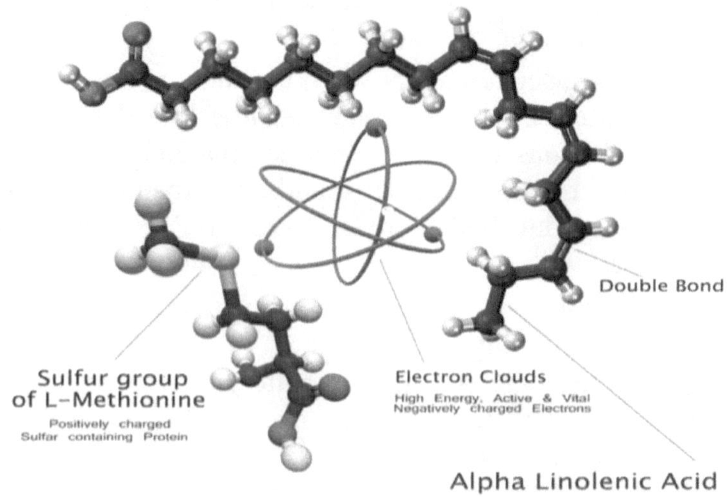

Dr. Budwig has been referred to as a top European cancer research scientist, biochemist, pharmacologist, and physicist. Dr. Budwig was a seven-time Nobel Prize nominee.

In Germany in 1952, she was the central government's senior expert for fats and pharmaceutical drugs. She's considered one of the world's leading authorities on fats and oils. Her research has shown the tremendous effects that commercially processed fats and oils (having Trans fatty acids) have in destroying cell membranes and lowering the voltage in the cells of our bodies, which then result in chronic and terminal disease including cancer.

What we have forgotten is that we are body electric. The cells of our body fire electrically. They have a nucleus in the center of the cell which is positively charged, and the cell membrane, which is the outer lining of the cell, is negatively charged. We are all aware of how fats clog up our veins and arteries and are the leading cause of heart attacks, but we never looked beyond the end of our noses to see how these very dangerous fats and oils are affecting the overall health of our minds and bodies at the cellular level.

Dr. Budwig discovered that when unsaturated fats have been chemically treated, their unsaturated qualities are destroyed and the field of electrons removed. This commercial processing of fats destroys the field of electrons that the cell membranes (60-75 trillion cells) in our bodies must have to fire properly (i.e. function properly).

The fats' ability to associate with protein and thereby to achieve water solubility in the fluids of the living body is destroyed. As Budwig put it, "the battery is dead because the electrons in these fats and oils recharge it." When the electrons are destroyed the fats are no longer active and cannot flow into the capillaries and through the fine capillary networks. This is when circulation problems arise.

Without the proper metabolism of fats in our bodies, every vital function and every organ is affected. This includes the generation of new life and new cells. Our bodies produce over 500 million new cells daily. Dr. Budwig points out that in growing new cells, there is a polarity between the electrically positive nucleus and the electrically negative cell membrane with its high unsaturated fatty acids. During cell division, the cell, and new daughter cell must contain enough electron-rich fatty acids in the cell's surface area to divide off completely from the old cell. When this process is interrupted the body begins to die. In essence, these commercially processed fats and oils are shutting down the electrical field of the cells allowing chronic and terminal diseases to take hold of our bodies.

A very good example would be tumors. Dr. Budwig noted that "The formation of tumors usually happens as follows. In those body areas which normally host many growth processes, such as in the skin and membranes, the glandular organs, for example, the liver and pancreas or the glands in the stomach and intestinal tract—it is here that the growth processes are brought to a standstill. Because the polarity is missing, due to the lack of electron rich highly unsaturated fat, the course of growth is disturbed—the surface-active fats are not present; the substance becomes inactive before the maturing and shedding process of the cells ever takes place, which results in the formation of tumors."

She pointed out that this can be reversed by providing the simple foods, cottage cheese, and flax seed oil, which revises the stagnated growth processes. This naturally causes the tumor or tumors present to dissolve and the whole range of symptoms which indicate a "dead battery are cured." Dr. Budwig did not believe in the use of growth-inhibiting treatments such as chemotherapy or radiation. She was quoted as saying "I flat declare that the usual hospital treatments today, in a case of tumorous growth, most certainly leads to worsening of the disease or a speedier death, and in healthy people, quickly causes cancer."

Dr. Budwig discovered that when she combined flaxseed oil, with its powerful healing nature of essential electron rich unsaturated fats, and cottage cheese, which is rich in sulfur protein, the bonding produced makes the oil water soluble and easily absorbed into the cell membrane.

I found testimonials of people from around the world who had been diagnosed with terminal cancer (all types of cancer), sent home to die and were now living healthy, normal lives. Not only had Dr. Budwig been using her protocol for treating cancer in Europe, but she also treated other chronic diseases such as arthritis, heart infarction, irregular heartbeat, psoriasis, eczema (other skin diseases), immune deficiency syndromes (Multiple Sclerosis and other autoimmune diseases), diabetes, lungs (respiratory conditions), stomach ulcers, liver, prostate, strokes, brain tumors, brain (strengthens activity), arteriosclerosis and other chronic diseases. Dr. Budwig's protocol proved successful where orthodox traditional medicine was failing.

Prime Cause of Cancer

We are fighting with cancer since the dawn of history. Every year we discover new diagnostic modalities, better radiotherapy techniques and lots of new chemotherapy drugs. But we have completely failed to defeat this disease called cancer. Think again, are we really going on the right path? Does conventional Medicine really targets upon the prime cause of cancer???

Otto Warburg – Biography

Otto Heinrich Warburg (October 8, 1883 – August 1, 1970), son of physicist Emil Warburg, was a German physiologist, medical doctor and Nobel laureate. His mother was the daughter of a Protestant family of bankers and civil servants from Baden. Warburg studied chemistry under the great Emil Fischer, and earned his "Doctor of Chemistry" in Berlin in 1906. He then earned the degree of "Doctor of Medicine" in Heidelberg in 1911. Between 1908 and 1914, Warburg was affiliated with the Naples Marine Biological Station, in Naples, Italy, where he conducted research.

He served as an officer in the elite Uhlan (cavalry regiment) during the First World War, and was given the Iron Cross (1st Class) award for his bravery. Warburg is considered one of the 20th century's leading biochemists. Towards the end of the war, Albert Einstein, who had been a friend of Warburg's father Emil, wrote Warburg asking him to leave the army and return to academia, since it would be a tragedy for the world to lose his talents. Einstein and Warburg later became friends, and Einstein's work in physics had great influence on Otto's biochemical research.

While working at the Marine Biological Station, Warburg performed research on oxygen consumption in sea urchin eggs after fertilization, and proved that upon fertilization, the rate of respiration increases by as much as six fold. His experiments also proved that iron is essential for the development of the larval stage.

In 1918, Warburg was appointed professor at the Kaiser Wilhelm Institute for Biology in Berlin-Dahlem. By 1931 he was promoted as director of the Kaiser Wilhelm Institute for Cell Physiology, which was later on, renamed the Max Planck Society. Warburg investigated the metabolism of tumors and the respiration of cells, particularly cancer cells, and in 1931 was awarded the Nobel Prize in Physiology for his "discovery of the nature and mode of action of the respiratory enzyme."

Nomination for a second Nobel Prize

In 1944, Warburg was nominated for a second Nobel Prize in Physiology by Albert Szent-Györgyi, for his work on nicotinamide, the mechanism and enzymes involved in fermentation, and the discovery of flavin (in yellow enzymes), but was prevented from receiving it by Adolf Hitler's regime.

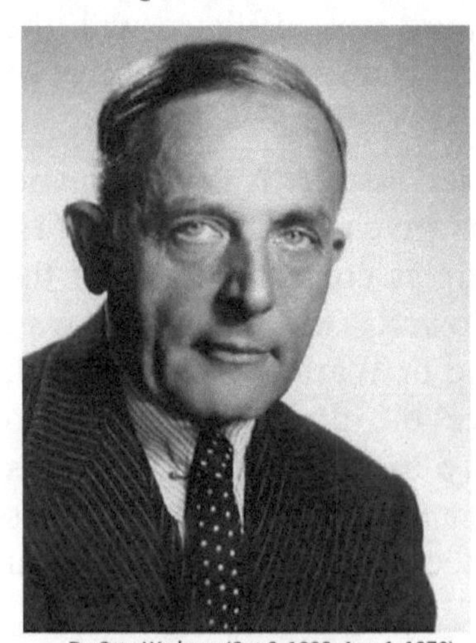
Dr. Otto Warburg (Oct 8, 1883 Aug 1, 1970)

Otto Warburg edited and had much of his original work published in The Metabolism of Tumors and wrote New Methods of Cell Physiology (1962). Otto Warburg was thrilled when Oxford University awarded him an honorary doctorate.

In his later years, Warburg was convinced that illness is resulted from pollution; this caused him to become a bit of a health advocate. He insisted on eating bread made from wheat grown organically on his farm. When he visited restaurants, he often made arrangements to pay the full price for a cup of tea, but to only be served boiling water, from which he would make tea with a tea bag he had brought with him. He was also known to go to significant lengths to obtain organic butter, the quality of which he trusted.

The Otto Warburg Medal

The Otto Warburg Medal is intended to commemorate Warburg's outstanding achievements. It has been awarded by the German Society for Biochemistry and Molecular Biology since 1963. The prize honors and encourages pioneering achievements in fundamental biochemical and molecular biological research. The Otto Warburg Medal is regarded as the highest award for biochemists and molecular biologists in Germany.

Prime cause of Cancer

Warburg hypothesized that cancer growth is caused by tumor cells mainly generating energy (as e.g. adenosine triphosphate / ATP) by anaerobic breakdown of glucose (known as fermentation, or anaerobic respiration). This is in contrast to healthy cells, which mainly generate energy from oxidative breakdown of pyruvate. Pyruvate is an end product of glycolysis, and is oxidized within the mitochondria. Hence, and according to Warburg, cancer should be interpreted as a mitochondrial dysfunction.

In short, Warburg summarized that all normal cells absolutely require oxygen, but cancer cells can live without oxygen - a rule without exception. Deprive a cell 35% of its oxygen for 48 hours and it would become cancerous. **Dr. Otto Warburg clearly mentioned that the root cause of cancer is lack of oxygen in the cells.**

He also discovered that cancer cells are anaerobic (do not breathe oxygen), get the energy by fermenting glucose and produce levo-rotating lactic acid, and the body becomes acidic.

Cancer cannot survive in the presence of high levels of oxygen, as found in an alkaline state.

He postulated that sulfur containing protein and some unknown fat is required to attract oxygen into the cell. This fat plays a major role in the respiration and functioning of Warburg respiratory enzyme. He thought it would be butyric acid and made experiment, but this attempt was a failure. For many decades scientists were trying to identify this unknown and mysterious fat but nobody succeeded (Otto Warburg, Wikipedia).

Dr. Johanna Budwig - Biography & Science

Birth of an angel

A lovely couple, Hermann Budwig and Elisabeth, lived in Essen town of Germany situated on the bank of river Ruhr. On the eve of 30th September, 1908 Elisabeth delivered a brilliant and lucky angel. Hermann and

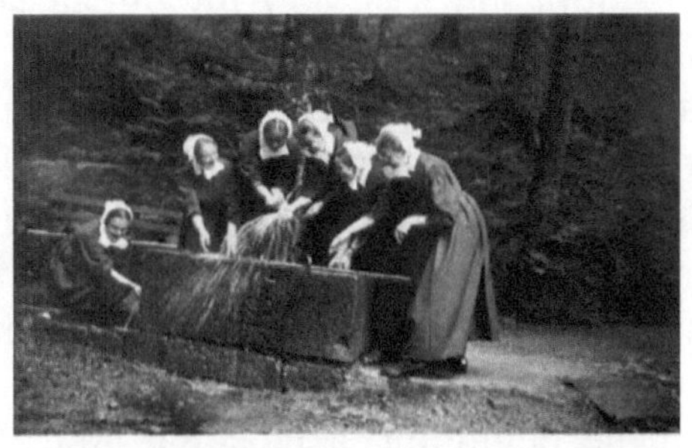

Elisabeth were very happy, and celebrating. They called her Johanna. In German, Johanna means a gift from God. In the family and neighborhood everybody was talking that Johanna is very lucky, she will study in a college and become a big doctor. Actually, 1908 was very fortunate and important year for the freedom of women in Germany. Government for the first time in history, changed laws, and allowed women to study in college and Universities. Also the German parliament passed a legislation to allow women to become members of political parties and prestigious clubs. Though women were given new rights and freedom, liberalization was slow and old values still persisted.

The tough life of a sage of science

Unluckily, Elisabeth died in 1920; family members thought that her father, being a poor loco mechanic, might not look after Johanna. So she was sent to an orphanage. This was a great shock for the little Johanna, but it had one positive side also. Education up to higher level was totally free for orphans.

In 1926, Germany was slowly recovering from the after effects of the First World War. Economic conditions were improving. Scholars and scientists were developing new technologies in every field. One third of all Nobel Prizes were being given to German academics.

Deaconess at Kaiserswerth

Johanna was very intelligent and sharp in studies from the beginning. In order to achieve good future, she decided to join the renowned Deaconess's Institute of Kaiserswerth in 1925. Theodor Fliedner, a pastor, founded Kaiserswerth Institute for welfare of unmarried mothers, prisoners, patients, orphans and poor children in 1836. In the beginning a Hospital and a Nursing School was established. This school was very famous Nursing School of that time. 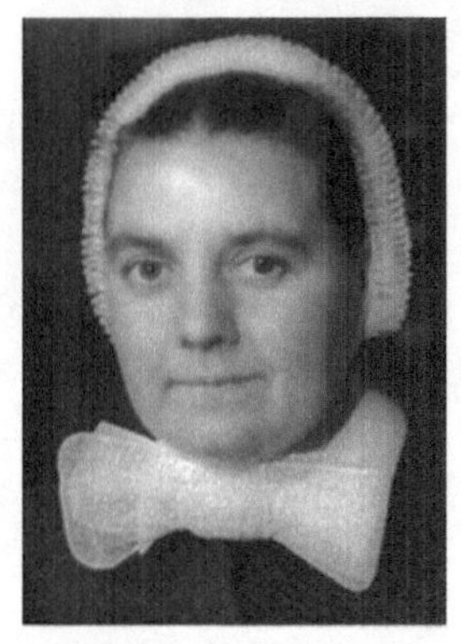 Florence Nightingale, known as mother of modern nursing, also studied in this Deaconess School in 1850. Intelligent Johanna easily got admission in this Institute. She was made a "deaconess" on March 30, 1932. This was the most appropriate place for her. There was a 1000 bedded hospital, pharmacy and a boarding school. She decided to study pharmacy.

After completing preliminary education in Kaiserswerth, she joined Münster University for further studies. Her analytical thinking and precise knowledge was noticed by her Professor Dr Hans Paul Kaufmann. He always encouraged and helped her. Here she passed state examination in pharmacy and was rewarded distinction in chemistry in 1936. Then she continued further education in physics, and received the title "Doctor of Science" at the University of Münster in 1938. On August 1, 1939, she was appointed as in-charge of pharmacy at the Military Hospital in Kaiserswerth.

Next month, Hitler's military forces attacked Poland. During war time, brave Johanna was busy in organizing and expanding the pharmacy. The war was not an easy time. There were two thousand people living in Kaiserswerth. Johanna was responsible for ensuring that there were enough medicines in this time of rationing and a thriving black market. She was well prepared and ready to fulfill any emergency demand for her patients. Many of her fellow deaconesses were often jealous and not co-operating but she continued evolving her professional skills. She was strong and was confronting every opponent (Dr. Johanna Budwig Stiftung).

Dr Budwig's scientific thinking, work and career

After Second World War, Johanna left Kaiserswerth in 1949. Soon Prof. Kaufmann came to know that she had left Kaiserswerth. He immediately met and persuaded her to work with him in Münster University, as he was always impressed from her talent. He converted the basement of his house into a laboratory and arranged all facilities for her research. He was famous as Fat Pope in the whole Europe.

On Prof. Kaufmann's recommendation, Johanna was appointed as the chief expert

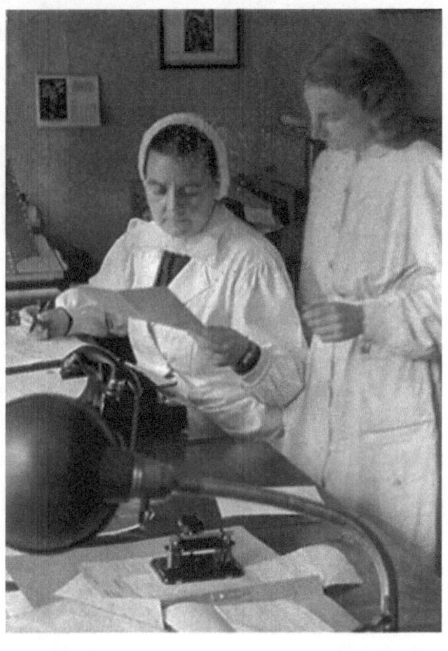

for drugs and fats at the Federal Institute for Fats Research, Germany. This was the country's largest office issuing the approval of new drugs used for cancer. Many applications had been submitted to her for approval. These were the medications for cancer therapy with the sulfhydryl group (sulfur-containing protein compounds). Everywhere she saw that fats played a role in cellular respiration, also in expert reports provided by well-known professors like Prof. Nonnenbruch. Unfortunately, fats could only be detected in the late stage, and there were no method to distinguish between fats chemically.

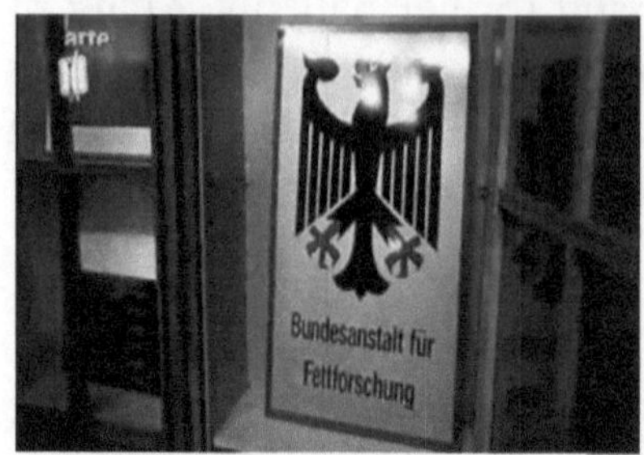

By this time, she developed paper chromatography. With this technique for first time she was able to detect fatty acids and lipoproteins directly even in 0.1 ml of blood. She used Co60 isotopes successfully to produce the first differential reaction for fatty acids, and produced the first direct iodine value via radioiodine. She also developed control of atmosphere in a closed system by using gas systems which act as antioxidants. She further developed Coloring methods, separating effects of fats and fatty acids. She too studied their behavior in blue and red light with fluorescent dyes.

Using rhodamine red dye, she studied the electrical behavior of the unsaturated fatty acids with their "halo". With this technique she could prove that electron rich highly unsaturated Linoleic and Linolenic fatty acids (Flax oil being the richest source) were the mysterious and undiscovered decisive fats required to attract oxygen into the cells, which Otto Warburg could not find. She studied the electromagnetic function of pi-electrons of the linolenic acid in the cell membranes, for nerve function, secretions, mitosis, as well as cell division. She also examined the synergism of the sulfur containing protein with the pi-electrons of the highly unsaturated fatty acids and their significance for the formation of the hydrogen bridge between fat and protein, which represent "the only path" for fast and focused Transport of electrons during respiration. This research was extensively

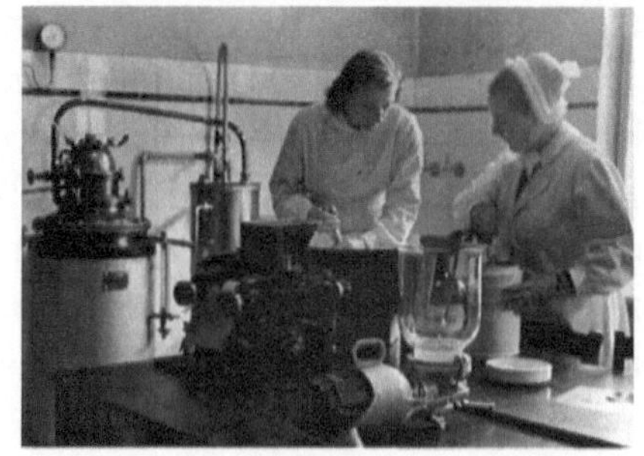

98

published in 1950 in Neue Wege in der Fettforschung (New Directions in Fat Research) and other publications.

This immediately caused an excitement and turmoil in the scientific community. Everybody thought that it would open new doors in Cancer research. She also proved that hydrogenated fats and refined oils including all Trans-fatty acids were not having vital electrons and were respiratory poisons.

During her research, she found that the blood of seriously ill cancer patients had deficiency of unsaturated essential fats (Linoleic and Linolenic fatty acids), lipoproteins, phosphatides, and hemoglobin. She also had noticed that cancer 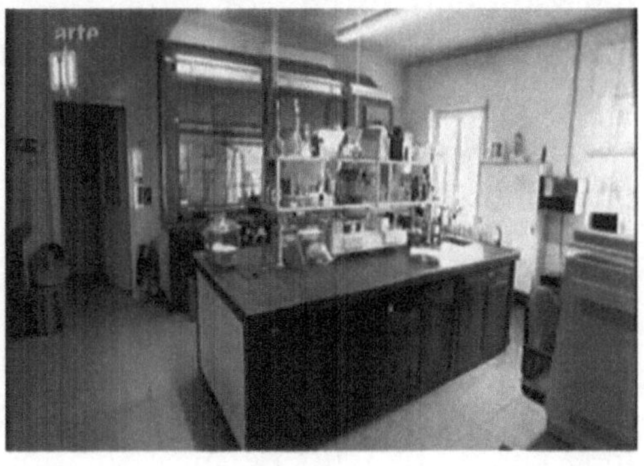 patients had a strange greenish-yellow substance in their blood which is not present in the blood of healthy people (Budwig, Cancer The Problem And The Solution).

She wanted to develop a healing program for cancer. So she enrolled over 642 cancer patients from four hospitals in Münster. She gave Flax oil and Cottage Cheeseto these patients. After just three months, patients began to improve in health and strength, the yellow green substance in their blood began to disappear, tumors gradually receded and at the same time the nutrients began to rise.

This way she developed a simple cure for cancer, based on the consumption of Flax oil with low fat Quark or cottage cheese, raw organic diet, mild exercise, Flax oil massage and the healing powers of the sun. It was a great victory and the first milestone in the battle against cancer. She treated approx. 2500 cancer patients during last few decades. Prof. Halme of surgery clinic in Helsinki used to keep records of her patients. According to him her success was over 90%, and this was achieved in cases, which were rejected by Allopathic doctors.

Dr. Budwig was a courageous scientist. She **loudly and convincingly argued that consumption of highly processed foods, particularly edible oils and margarines, which block the oxidation processes in the cells, are responsible for the development of cancer and other degenerative diseases.** She met with great resistance from food industry giants, who were doing everything to prevent the spread of her sensational discovery. In 1952, under the influence of strong pressure from this lobby, she lost her job and was barred from the research work.

Joins Medical School at Göttingen

Opponents of Dr. Johanna blamed her that she should not treat cancer patients because she doesn't have a doctor's degree. She felt this and eventually joined medical school in Göttingen in

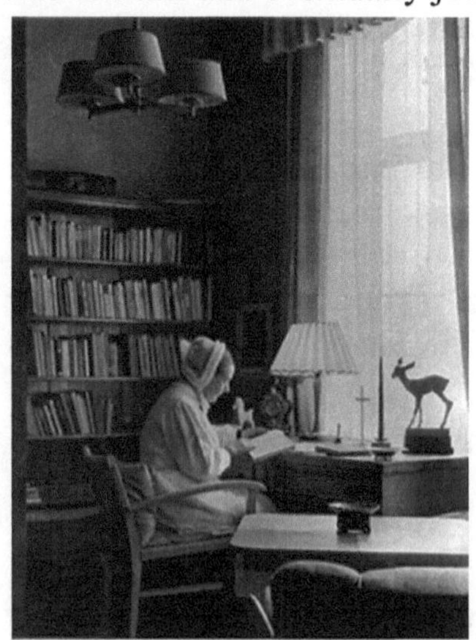

1955. Budwig was 47 years old at that time. She also continued her research work along with her studies. *Budwig successfully treated Prof. Martius's wife, who suffered from Breast Cancer*

One night a woman came with her small child whose arm was supposed to be amputated due to a tumor. She treated her and soon the amputation surgery was dismissed, and the child quickly did very well.

A Swiss woman came to her clinic in Göttingen. She suffered from Colon Cancer with metastasis and intestinal obstruction. Several doctors examined her, and were to be operated on Christmas Eve. On Budwig's request, she was treated by her protocol. The tumor of the colon quickly subsided. Seven weeks later, she was discharged without any detectable tumor. It is interesting that the Swiss custom officer was not ready to believe that the submitted passport belonged to same lady. Her look was so much changed! At home her daughter welcomed saying: "You look healthy, younger and more beautiful (from her book The Death of the Tumor – Vol. II).

After this, University allowed her to treat cancer patients with her oil-protein diet. She was getting miraculous results. University professors were excited with the results, but wanted that she should also include chemo and radiotherapy. She was rigid and didn't want to compromise. So she had differences and conflicts with her professors and ultimately left Göttingen (Budwig, Cancer The Problem And The Solution).

Last Destination - Dietersweiler-Freudenstadt

Eventually, she shifted to Dietersweiler-Freudenstadt, where she lived till her death. There she completed Ph.D. in Naturopathy so that she could legally treat cancer patients. She continued treating her patients in Freudenstadt. In 1968 she created unique Eldi oils for massage and enema, called Electron Differential Oils after performing precise spectroscopic measurements of the light absorption in different oils. *US pain institute has written somewhere: "What this crazy woman does with her ELDI oils, none of us manages to do via pain killers."*

Budwig conducted more than 200 lectures worldwide. Dr. Budwig was popular in the U.S. as FLAX SEED lady from Freudenstadt. She delivered her last public Lecture in Freudenstadt on March 3, 1999. On November 28, 2002, she fell down in her bathroom and got a fracture in right femur neck. She was admitted in a nursing home and ultimately died on May 19, 2003.

Budwig Protocol

The Budwig Protocol is one of the most widely followed alternative treatments for cancer and other diseases. The diet seems simple, but foods are powerful and can heal a person.

Transition Diet

The Transition diet is especially recommended for patients of liver, pancreatic or gall bladder cancers. The basic principle is that for 3 days nothing is eaten and drunk except the following written and at least three times daily warm tea (herbal teas from peppermint, rose hip, mallow or green tea) is drunk. Dr Budwig has recommended variant 1 for patients with a relatively good energy state, and variant 2 and 3 mainly for seriously ill patients.

Variant 1

Variant 1 for three days, 250 g of linomel or alternatively freshly crushed Flax seed is eaten together with the following:

- Freshly pressed fruit juices without added sugar.
- Freshly pressed vegetable juices such as carrot, celery juice, red beetroots and apple juice.
- Chinese tea and black tea are allowed in the morning
- Honey for sweetening is allowed. Just as grape juice for drinking and as a sweetener. Energetically weak patients can also consume sparkling wine and linomel.

Variant 2

For three days, oat meal cereal very hour with linomel is eaten daily with the following juices:

- Freshly pressed fruit juices or freshly pressed vegetable juices such as carrot, celery juice, beetroot and apple juice.
- Chinese tea and black tea are allowed in the morning.
- Honey for sweetening is allowed. Just as grape juice for drinking and as a sweetener.

- Energetically weak patients can also consume sparkling wine and linomel.

Variant 3

For three days, oatmeal soup with linomel is given three times a day together with the following juices:

- Freshly pressed fruit juices or fruit juices without added sugar.
- Freshly pressed vegetable juices such as carrot, celery juice, beetroot and apple juice.
- Chinese tea and black tea are allowed in the morning.
- Honey for sweetening is allowed. Just as grape juice for drinking and as a sweetener.
- Energetically weak patients can also consume sparkling wine and linomel.

It is often experienced frequently that patients mixed all three variants and "nevertheless" had good results. So better you to stick to one variant. (Budwig – Cancer The Problem And The Solution 2005: p.36).

Budwig Diet

The Budwig Protocol is necessary for many diseases from cancer to type 2 diabetes and heart disease to autoimmune diseases, etc. Its purpose is to energize the cells by restoring the natural electrical potential in the cell. Many human diseases are caused by "sick cells" which have lost their normal electrical potential; generally via a lower ATP energy in the cell's mitochondria.

6:00 AM – Sauerkraut juice

A glass of sauerkraut juice consumed before breakfast every morning. It is rich in vitamins including C, enzymes and helps develop the health-promoting gut flora. Sauerkraut is cabbage that has been pickled by natural fermentation, mainly with lactobacillus bacteria. It is slightly salty, sharp and sour. Well made, it is much nicer than it sounds. You may also consume another glass of sauerkraut juice later in the day.

It interesting that sauerkraut contains right rotating lactic acids and is highly alkaline and neutralizes levo-rotating lactic acids and makes our body alkaline. That is why Marcus Porcius Cato the Elder issued a statement - Carcinomas are incurable except with the treatment with Sauerkraut.

8:00 AM Breakfast

Green or herbal tea

Start breakfast with a cup of warm herbal or green tea. Sweeten with only natural honey. You can add lemon or grape juice. Patient should take such a tea before or with Linomel Muesli. You may consume 4-5 such teas in a day.

Linomel Muesli or Oil-Protein Muesli

This should be made fresh and consumed within 15 minutes.

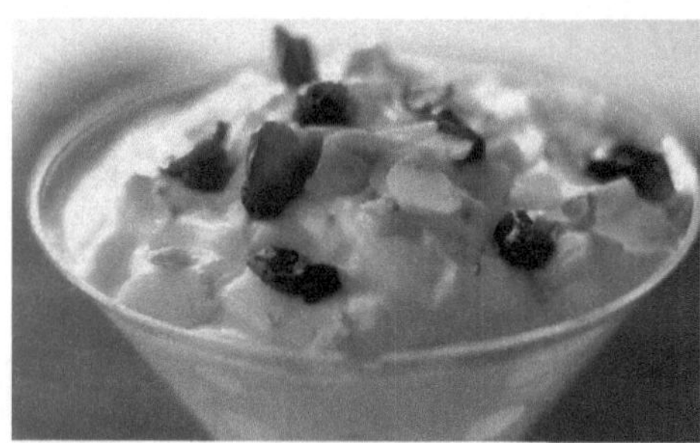

It is full of high energy pi-electrons, attract oxygen in the cells and capable of healing cell membranes. It is full of energy-rich omega-3 fats, has power to attract healing photons from sun through resonance. As "Om" is divine word and synonym of God in India. According to Hindu Mythology, the whole universe is located inside "Om", so the name Omkhand has been given to this wonderful recipe in Hindi.

Ingredients

- 3 Tbsp cold pressed organic Flax seed oil (FO)
- 100-125gm (6 Tbsp) Quark or Cottage Cheese(CC)
- 2 Tbsp freshly ground Flax seeds
- 2 Tbsp milk

- 1 cup fruits
- ¼ cup dried nuts
- Natural honey
- Flavorings – lemon, apple cider vinegar, cinnamon, pure cacao, natural vanilla, shredded coconut etc.

Recipe

Place 2 tablespoons Linomel or freshly ground Flax seeds in a small bowl. It is covered with raw, crushed or diced seasonal fruits depending on the season. Pour some orange or grape juice over this. Linomel^{Tm} is a brand name and originally created and patented by Budwig. It is a cereal made from cracked Flax Seed, a small amount of honey and a little milk powder.

Then the Quark-Flax seed oil cream is prepared in as follows: First add Flax seed oil, milk and honey and blend briefly with a hand-held immersion electric blender, then gradually add the Quark in smaller portions. Blend till oil and Quark is thoroughly mixed with no separated oil. Then it is seasoned differently everyday with different flavorings such as vanilla, cinnamon or various fruits such as banana, apple, lemon, orange juice, or berries.

Use various fruits such as fresh berries, apple, cherry, orange, banana, papaya, grapes etc. Add other fresh fruit if you like, totaling ½ to 1 cup of fruit. Budwig specially advised to use berries like strawberry, blueberry, raspberry, cheery

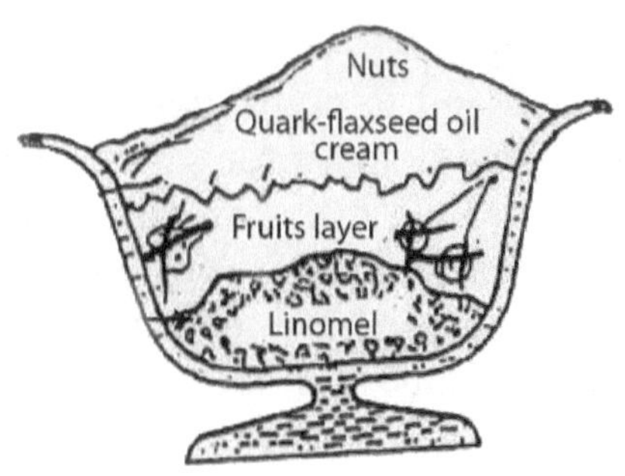

etc. because berries have ellagic acids which are strong cancer fighters.

Add organic raw nuts such as walnuts, almonds, raisins or Brazil nuts. They have sulfurated proteins, omega-3 fats and vitamins. Brazil nut is especially important because a single nut provides you with all of the selenium you need for the day. Selenium is very important to boost immune power. Peanuts are prohibited.

For variety and flavor, try natural vanilla, cinnamon, lemon juice, pure cocoa or shredded coconut.

Once blended in Budwig Cream, Quark and Flax seed oil form a new substance called lipoprotein. Lipoprotein is a water soluble complex. The Quark is rich in the sulfur-containing amino acids, methionine and cysteine. These positively charged amino acids attract the negatively charged electron clouds in fatty acid chains and exhibit a stabilizing effect on the highly unsaturated, otherwise easily oxidized fats. Thus, the amino acids protect the polyunsaturated fatty acids from the Flax seed oil against oxidation which, as a result, are able to enter the human body unchanged and with their full energy potential. The result: they are much more valuable to cells and their membranes. Consequently, one could say that Quark excels as a protector for the polyunsaturated fatty acids.

Sulfur-rich amino acids play a wealth of roles in many vital functions in our bodies. In combination with polyunsaturated fatty acids, they are important partners in regulating the uptake of oxygen and its utilization by the cell. They therefore contribute significantly to a strong immune system, healthy metabolism, and mental vitality. For many generations, people have been getting their omega-3 fatty acids from fish, vegetables, nuts, and seeds. Our health literally depends on the regular consumption of the essential omega-3 and omega-6 fatty acids, alpha-linolenic acid (ALA) and linoleic acid (LA). Our bodies require these fatty acids in order to synthesize their cell membranes as well as for a variety of metabolic processes and heal the cancer and other diseases.

Tips for making the Budwig Mixture

- Follow directions properly! It is important to add things to the mixture in the right order. If you mix them in the wrong order you may lose a lot of the opportunity to convert the oil-soluble omega-3 into water soluble-omega-3.
- Keep the Flax seed oil refrigerated.
- Immersion blender is a must.
- The mixture can be flavored differently every day by adding nuts and fruits preferably organic such as pecans, almonds or walnuts (not peanuts), banana, organic cocoa, shredded coconut, pineapple (fresh) blueberries, raspberries, cinnamon, vanilla or (freshly) squeezed fruit juice.
- Consume immediately for best results.

10 AM Vegetable juice

Freshly squeezed vegetable juice from carrots, beets, celery, tomato, and radish, lemon as well as green vegetables - stinging nettle, lettuce or spinach. Apple is added to sweeten and enhance the taste. Carrot & beet juices are especially helpful to the liver and have strong cancer fighting properties. Vary vegetables. Some tasty and nutritious combinations are beet and apple juice, carrot and apple, carrot and beet, asparagus and apple, celery and apple, celery and carrot. Beet juice should not be taken alone. If taken alone it may cause red or pink urine (beeturia).

She also frequently recommended the following juices:

1. Nettle juice - Especially in the spring, Dr Budwig recommended to puree nettles with water and a lemon.

2. Radish juice - For this, a radish is first crushed and then thrown together with a lemon into the juicer. This juice is by the way durable for several days and Dr Budwig has sometimes recommended her patients to drink a small quantity of them every day.

3. Coltsfoot juice - For this juice, with the exception of the harder old rootstock, the entire remaining underground shoot is mixed with a few flowers and some milk and honey.

4. Horseradish juice - Mix 3-5 cm horseradish together with an apple and (raw) milk. Depending on the quantity of milk you can change the taste. Dr Budwig recommended this juice above all to workmen and to stimulate the appetite. Freshly pressed means, by the way, that you drink the juice within 5 minutes after pressing. In some cases, Dr Budwig prescribed a second juice 30 to 60 minutes later.

12:15 PM Lunch

Salad Platter: Salad plate with homemade cottage cheese-Flax seed mayonnaise. As salad also use: dandelion, cress, celery, tomato, cucumber, lettuce, radish, cabbage, broccoli, green horseradish and pepper.

Delicious mayo salad dressing can be prepared by mixing together 2 Tbsp (30 ml) Flax Oil, 2 Tbsp (30 ml) milk, and 2 Tbsp (30 ml) cottage cheese. Then add 2 tablespoons (30 ml) of Lemon juice (or Apple Cider Vinegar) and add 1 teaspoon (2.5 g) Mustard powder plus some herbs of your choice. Other alternative dressing can be made by mixing Flax Oil, lemon juice, Mustard and some herbs (Budwig, The Oil-Protein Diet Cookbook, 1994).

Main Course: Vegetables cooked in water, then flavored with Oleolox and herbs possibly with oatmeal, soy sauce, curry etc. Vegetable broth flavored with

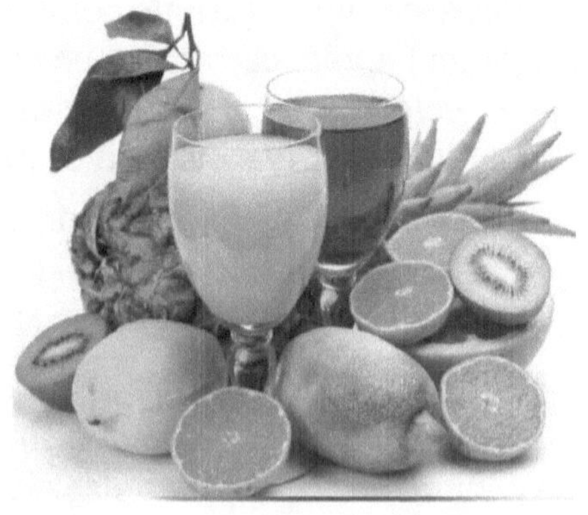

a little Oleolox and yeast flakes. As side dish for the vegetables: buckwheat, brown rice, millet or potatoes can be used. One or two slices of Ezekiel bread can be taken. Use lot of dried fruits in the main meal also.

Lunch Dessert: Cottage cheese/ Flax oil mixture served as a dessert, prepared with dry fruits and fruits such as apple, or poured over a fruit salad. You already know how to prepare it perfectly. You will find wonderful recipes for a delicious dessert in the Oil-Protein cookbook by Budwig. Please note that the dessert is **"a must"** and should definitely be eaten. So keep your main course light so you may enjoy the dessert happily.

The form of preparation as "fruit foam," "Linovita" or "red coat in the snow" (in Oil-Protein cookbook) is always welcoming for the healthy and the sick. In all the gimmicks in the preparation of the delicious desserts, one should be aware: Quark and Flaxseed give the patient immense power within a short space of time. Always fresh and beautiful, always freshly interesting, this important food for life should be for the sick and for the whole family.

3 PM Fruit juices

In the afternoon, Dr Budwig recommended different kinds of fruit juices e.g. apples, grapes, cherries, pineapples, papaya, or apricot, sparkling wine or wine - with or without Flaxseeds or with or without a few drops Flaxseed oil.

Budwig preferred papaya juice and recommended her patients to drink at least every 2 days a glass of papaya juice. The main reason for this was definitely the protein splitting enzyme papain.

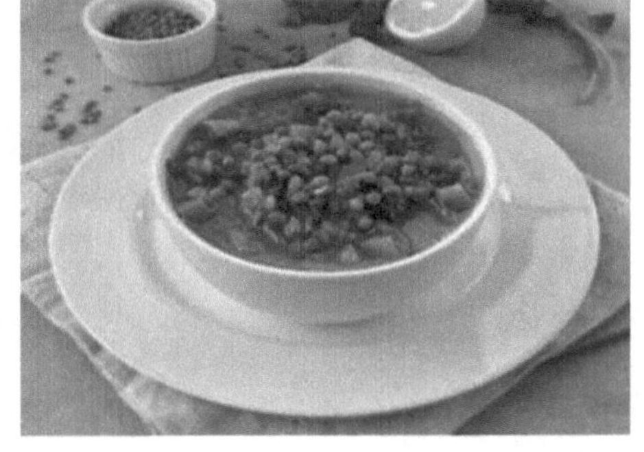

6 PM Dinner

The evening meal should be light and served early, around 6 p.m. A warm meal may be prepared using brown rice, buckwheat or oat meal. Never consume corn or soy beans. Dishes made with buckwheat grouts are most easily tolerated and nourishing. Use only honey to sweeten. Soup or more solid dishes can be combined with a tasty sauce according to preference. Use OLEOLOX liberally also to sweet sauces and soups, making them nourishing and a richer source of energy.

8:30 PM

A glass of organic red wine may be consumed. All things are a matter of correct dosage. This glass of red wine is not a "must" program. In fact, seriously ill patients having pain and discomfort just starting on the oil-protein diet, it is recommended to serve a glass of red wine mixed with freshly ground Flax seeds to tide them over while going off pain killers (Budwig, Cancer The Problem And The Solution).

METRIC CONVERSION TABLE	
10 g = 0.35 oz	5 cc = 1 teaspoon
100 g = 3.5 oz	15 cc = 1 tablespoon
150 g = 5.25 oz	30 cc = 1 ounce
250 g = 8.8 oz	250 cc = 1 cup
454 g = 1 lb	960 cc = 1 qt
Oz = ounce lb = pound qt = quart Tsp = teaspoon Tbsp = tablespoon	

Precautions

Drink filtered water - Use RO (Reverse Osmosis)water for drinking, cooking and enemas.

Eat Organic Diet - Always try to eat organic food.

Dental Care –

Mercury is a Carcinogenic as well as a Poison! The root canals of dead teeth are full of bacteria that attack the liver and lymphatic system. From Amalgam fillings the mercury slowly leaks out of the filings. The ADA cleverly defends the use of amalgam in spite of the fact that there is sufficient evidence that patients with many severe problems, including psychotic episodes and fatal allergic reactions, were just cured by removing the amalgam. It is advisable to rather have a ceramic filling than be slowly poisoned by mercury. Even gold filling is dangerous; it acts as battery producing electrical current. Be informed that the effect of drugs, including poison, is dose dependant and cumulative.

Fluoride is not only toxic but it is also carcinogenic. Fluoride has never been proven to prevent tooth decay. It has been outlawed in many countries or groups of countries because the evidence is overwhelming that fluoride causes premature aging, so drink bottled water and use fluoride-free toothpaste (American Cancer Institute - 1963).

I highly recommend helping you avoid fillings in the first place. Holistic dentist recommend 3% H_2O_2 as a gargle or rinse, or making a paste using baking soda. H_2O_2 usage three times a day is advised. It is great for cleaning dentures, too.

Frying and deep frying - Frying and deep frying is not allowed to cook patient's food. Never heat any oil in the kitchen. By heating oils the wealth of high energy electrons is destroyed and Trans fats and dangerous toxic chemicals such as acrylamides are formed in the oil. Boiling and steaming are good practices. You can fry vegetables etc. in water and add oleolox before

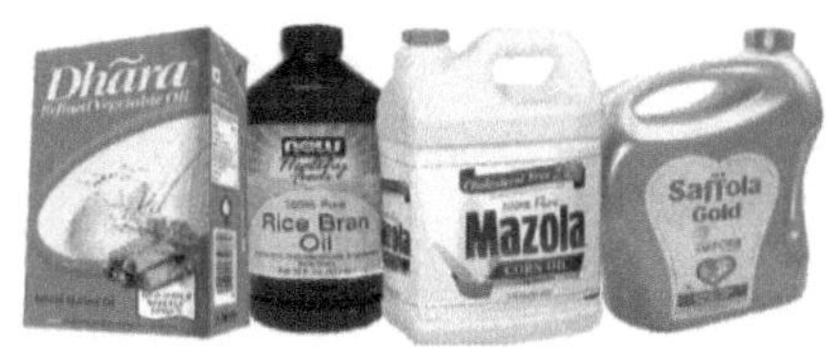

serving. Water is the safest medium for frying, says Lothar Hirneise.

Chemo and Radio -

Chemotherapy is aimed at destruction of the tumor, and it destroys many living cells, and the entire person. Anything that disturbs growth is fatal because growth is an elementary 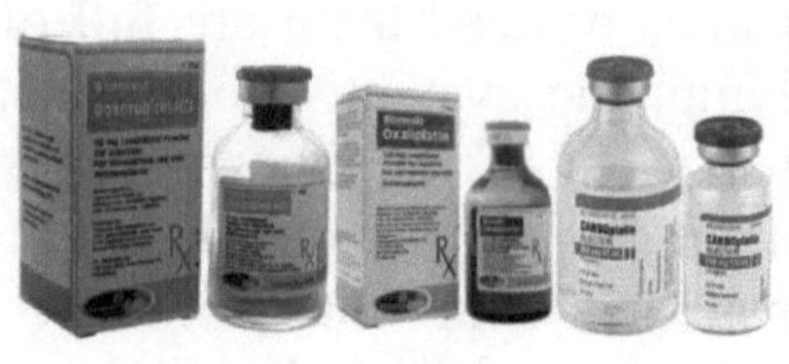 function of life. We cannot achieve something good with bad tools.

Dr. Budwig rejects Chemo and Radiation Therapy. Budwig used to say with full confidence and clarity, "My treatment targets on the real cause of cancer; it fills cancer cells with high energy pi-electrons and attracts oxygen into the cells. And cancer cells start to breathe and produce vital energy."

Man-made Supplements - With this treatment man-made antioxidants, synthetic vitamins and pain killers should not be given. The dose of anticoagulants and aspirin should be adjusted by your doctor. Dr. Budwig favors natural, herbal and homeopathy instead of man-made and synthetic supplements, vitamins and pain killers (Budwig, Cancer The Problem And The Solution).

Prohibitions of Budwig Protocol

In this protocol there are certain restrictions. They are as important as the diet itself. It is very difficult to defeat the cancer without strictly following these rules.

Sugar is strictly forbidden

Sugar, Jiggery, molasses, maple syrup and artificial sweeteners like xylitol, aspartame are not permitted. You can use only natural honey, stevia and fruit juices – all off course unprocessed.

Avoid meats, eggs and fish

Meat, fish, poultry, eggs, and butter are never allowed. Preserved meat is like a poison. It is highly processed and treated with dangerous antibiotics, preservatives and nitrates.

Stop using Hydrogenated Fat and Refined oil

You can never eat pizza, burger, fast food, fried food, biscuits etc. as they all are made by hydrogenated margarine and shortenings. Hydrogenation is a very dangerous process, used to increase shelf life of fats. In this process (oil is heated at very high temperature and hydrogen is passed through oils in presence of nickel) killing Trans fats are formed, high energy live and vital electrons are destroyed and nutrients are damaged. Hydrogenated Fats is just a dead, nutrition-less and cancer causing liquid plastic. Budwig always preached against these damaging fats. She has allowed low fat cheese, oleolox and coconut oil.

Preservatives and Processed Food

You should not eat Potato chips, soft drinks etc. which are full of preservatives. Never consume highly processed food e.g. ready to eat packed foods, pasta, pastries, bread and soy products, tofu etc. However good quality soy souse is permitted.'

Microwave, Teflon, Aluminum and Plastic

Never cook in microwave oven. Food cooked in microwave become toxic and deformed. Also don't use aluminum, plastic, Teflon coated cookware and aluminum foils. Use stainless steel, iron, china clay or glass utensils instead.

Chemicals and pesticides are not allowed

Avoid pesticides and chemicals, even those in household products & cosmetics. Stay away from mosquito repellants, sun screen lotions and sun glasses.

Wear natural fibers

Don't wear clothes made using synthetic fiber like nylon, polyester and acrylic. Budwig put great emphasis on the fact that her patients only wore natural fabrics such as cotton or satin, since they too can influence the magnetic field of our body.

Bed

Don't use on foam pillow and mattress. She recommended horsehair mattresses. Latex mattresses are the second choice. In any case, however, you should always replace mattresses that have metal spring cores.

CRT TV and mobile phones

These emit dangerous electromagnetic radiation, so do not use them. You can watch LCD and plasma TVs.

No left over

Food should be prepared fresh and eaten soon after preparation to maximize intake of health giving electrons and enzymes (Budwig, Cancer The Problem And The Solution).

Fujiya delight

Ingredients for 3 people:
> 250 cc grape juice, 250 cc pure currant juice,
> 8g agar-agar, Quark-Flaxseed oil,
> Milk, honey, vanilla cream

Preparation:

Heat the grape juice till it boils, then add the currant juice, agar-agar, stirring constantly for 5 minutes, and allow to cool. Now divide this mass to 3 narrow, tall cups, which have been rinsed with cold water. It is preferable if these cups have a bottom diameter of only 3- 4 cm. Refrigerate to cool. Now mix a Quark-Flaxseed oil cream with milk, honey and vanilla. Turn the red jelly upside down onto glass plates. The Quark-Flaxseed oil cream is placed on the top so that only the upper half is covered with the Quark-Flaxseed oil cream, so that top looks like the Snow caped Mount Fujiyama.

(The beautiful hotel with a gorgeous view of the Fujiyama is called "Fujiya", hence the dessert "Fujiya".)

Linovita-in-love in wine jelly

Ingredients: for 5 people:
> 250 cc of grape juice, 250 ccm of white wine,
> 8 agar-agar, 4 tablespoons of milk,
> 8 tablespoons of Flaxseed oil, 2 teaspoons of honey,
> 200-250 g of Quark, 2 liqueur glasses
> Vodka, plum (Slibowitz) or cherry brandy or rum

Preparation:

The wine jelly is prepared by heating 250 cc of grape juice till it boils. Agar-agar is stirred with a little wine and placed in the boiling grape juice. Immediately remove from the cooking plate and add the remaining wine gradually with constant stirring. After about 5 minutes, the jelly mixture clears itself. You can now divide to approx. 5 glass bowls or champagne glasses. Immediately afterwards, mix the Quark-Flaxseed oil cream from Flaxseed oil, milk, honey and Quark. Finally, add 2 liqueur glasses of vodka or slibovitz or cherry brandy or rum into the Quark-Flaxseed oil cream. This Quark-Flaxseed oil mixture is evenly divided on the ready to-use bowls so that the Quark-Flaxseed oil cream partly sinks down in the middle. It is served after complete solidification.

Ice cream with cocoa

Ingredients:
>   3 tablespoons of Flaxseed oil, 3 tablespoons of milk,
>   1 tablespoon of honey, 100g of Quark, 100 g of hazelnuts,
>   2 tablespoons of cocoa

Preparation:
Quark, Flaxseed oil, milk and honey are mixed in the blender, then the hazelnuts are added, well blended and finally, cocoa is added to the mixture. Now pour the entire mixture into the ice-maker and place it in the fridge compartment of the refrigerator. This mixture with a nougat flavor gives the various combinations mentioned here the dark color contrasts. For very ill people these preparations are very important, especially when there is a general lack of appetite.

> (Oil-Protein Diet by Lothar Hirneise *available at*
> *http://www.hirneise.com/page-8/page-19/)*

ELDI oils

Dr. Budwig created unique ELDI oils, called electron differential oils after performing precise spectroscopic measurements of the light absorption in different oils - specifying that the oils contained pi-electron clouds from Flax oil, wheat germ oil plus vitamin-E in its natural complex, etheric oils and sulfhydryl groups.

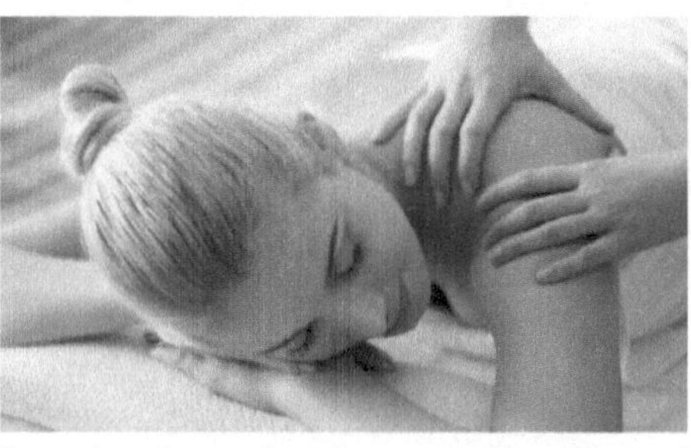

Dr. Johanna Budwig said, "The sun is my preferred treatment modality, as is ELDI oil, used externally to stimulate the absorption of the long-wave band of the sun. I have used ELDI oils extensively since 1968 for body massage as well as in the selective application of oil packs. US pain institute has written somewhere: "What this crazy woman does with her ELDI oils, none of us manages to do via pain killers." Dr. Budwig has mentioned that if ELDI oil is not available, you may use Flax oil instead. *You can buy ELDI oils at: www.sensei.de*

Massage Benefits

- Since ancient time massage has been part of cancer healing. Think of your lymphatics as a trash-disposal system for your body. Massage initiates lymphatic drainage, you push the trash out of your body and you're helping your immune system.
- Massage therapy is sometimes the first really pleasant touch a patient is able to experience.
- Massage also releases endorphins (our body's natural painkillers), stimulates lymph movement, and stretches

tissues throughout the body. It's energizing, stimulating, and pretty good feeling.

ELDI oil plans:

A: For cancer patients in support of the energy level

1. Full-body rubbings in the morning
2. ELDI oil R enema with 200ml every 2-3 days
3. Wrap at the "place of the happening"

B: For energetically weak patients
1. Full-body rubbings in the morning and in the evening
2. Enema: standard plan for ELDI oil R
3. Wrap at the "place of the happening"
4. Daily liver wrap with ELDI oil sage

Additional information:

- Make sure that you make once a week an (deep/high) enema with water or coffee.
- If you make daily coffee enemas, then start in the morning with the coffee enema and then with the ELDI R enema, but only if your energetic level allows you to make two enemas daily. Otherwise, only make the ELDI R enema. (Oil Protein Diet by Lothar Hirneise)

ELDI oils from SENSEI (www.sensei.de) are produced in a permanent cold chain in a European oil mill and marketed under the name of Electron Differentiation Oils. There are two qualities. A 6-star organic quality and a 5-star quality, which are produced exclusively for the IOPDF (www.iopdf.com).

Cost factor ELDI oils

Again and again we hear that for reasons of cost, patients use Flax seed oil instead of ELDI oil R for an enema. Please do not do so, because Flax seed oil does not react in the same way as ELDI oil R. Instead, use cheap ELDI oils from IOPDF or reduce the amount of oil.

Procedure –

Two times a day, i.e. morning and evening, rub ELDI Oil or Flax oil into the skin over the whole body, a bit more intensely on the shoulders, armpits and groin area (where plenty of lymphatic vessels are present) as well as the problem areas, such as the breast, stomach, liver, etc. Leave the oil on the skin for about 20 minutes and follow with a warm water shower without washing with soap. After 10 minutes take another shower, this time using a mild soap, and then relax for 15-20 minutes.

Once the body has been oiled and the ELDI Oil or Flax oil has penetrated the skin, the warm water will open the skin pores and the oil penetrates the skin more deeply. The second shower, where one washes with soap, cleanses the skin so that clothes and linen will not become overly soiled.

Oil Packs

Take a piece of cloth made of pure cotton. Cut to a size to fit the body part, such as the knee. Soak the cotton cloth with oil, place on the knee etc., cover it with a piece of polythene and wrap it up with an elastic bandage. Leave overnight. Remove in the morning and wash the knee; repeat in the evening. Keep applying the same procedure for weeks, you get good results. You also use Flax oil or castor oil for these local applications if you do not get ELDI oils . Dr Budwig generally recommended ELDI sage and should be used in the following indications:

- Tumors
- Painful skin areas
- Metastases
- Hepatic impairment and liver support
- Kidney problems
- Bladder disorders
- Intestinal cramps
- Lung disorders
- Bone disorders of all kinds

ELDI Oil Enema

Enemas are used in the Oil-Protein Diet exclusively for the energy intake and not for the purification of the intestine. Dr Budwig used to give ELDI oil or Flax oil enema to her serious patients. Budwig used to get immediate and miraculous results with the most seriously ill patients. Flax seed Oil enema also give similar results.

I recommend you to make the first enemas only with 100ml and then increase over several days to 250ml. Some patients have enemas with 500ml oil and positively reported on it. 500ml are however the absolute exception and mostly not necessary. Usually 250ml suffice.

Incidentally, smaller amounts are also easily introduced with an enema syringe instead of with an enema bucket. Enema syringes are available in sizes up to 350ml and are easy to handle.

Standard plan for ELDI oil R: Day 1 = 100ml, day 2 = 100ml, day 3 = 150ml, day 4 = 150ml, day 5 = 200ml, day 6 = 200ml and day 7 = 250ml.

From the seventh day, one remains at 250ml, and so long until the patient is significantly better. Then you can go back to 100ml - 150ml, always together with 1-2 daily whole body rubbings. (Oil Protein Diet by Lothar Hirneise)

Ingredients

- Enema pot
- Watch
- A bowl to collect oil when you are getting rid of bubbles.
- Towel and tissue
- RO filtered water
- ELDI oil or Flax oil
- Towel or Drip Stand

Procedure

Prepare a place near the toilet, so that if you can't hold the enema, you will be making a quick dash and the shorter distance is better.

Cleansing Enema with Plain water

First of all you should take a plain water enema. Purpose of this enema is cleaning of intestines. It is not a retention enema and is evacuated immediately. For this you may use 500-1000ml (2-4 cups) RO filtered water. As soon as the whole water is inside the rectum, go and sit on the commode and release the water slowly.

Take the oil enema immediately after the water enema

- Use advised (above) amount of ELDI or Flax oil. The oil should be at body temperature. The best test is to dip your little finger into the oil.
- Fill the oil into the enema pot. It takes at least 5 minutes for the bubbles to get out of the tube.
- The enema pot should be hanged on a drip stand about 2-3 feet above your body.
- You need to lubricate the nozzle and anus with Flax oil. When all is ready, lie on your right side in the fetal position. Insert the nozzle into the rectum slowly and carefully with your left hand, and un-pinch the tube.
- If you feel little uncomfortable when the oil is going in, pinch the tube, wait till the feeling passes away, then continue again.
- The oil is much more viscous and moves more slowly. You might need to hold the pot a bit higher to get it to run a bit quicker.
- Once the oil is in, wait and hold it for about 12 minutes. After that slowly turn yourself to left side and hold oil for

another 12 minutes. You may listen to music while taking enema.

- When done, it is best to sit on the commode for about 15 minutes with something to read (Skelton).

Coffee Enema

Dr. Max Gerson introduced coffee enema back in the 1930s. In this enema about 500ml of coffee is pushed into rectum, this amount only reaches up to sigmoid colon. There is no loss of minerals and electrolytes in Coffee Enema because their absorption occurs well before sigmoid colon. Coffee enema is even safe for those who are allergic to coffee because it is not absorbed into the systemic circulation. You may take this enema once or twice. It has the following benefits:

- **Powerful and Natural Pain Reliever**
- **Cleansing -** Coffee also acts as an astringent in the large intestine, helps cleanse the colon walls.
- **Toxin Elimination -** The major benefit of the coffee enema is elimination of toxins through the liver. Caffeine, theophylline and theobromine dilate the blood vessels and bile ducts, stimulate the liver to discharge more bile and boost the detoxifying process into high gear and heal inflammation. Indeed, endoscopic studies confirm they increase bile output.
- **Stimulates Liver -** Kahweol and cafestol palmitate found in coffee promote the activity of a key enzyme system called glutathione S-Transferase. This is an important mechanism in the detoxification of carcinogens, as the

enzyme group is responsible for neutralizing free radicals. Coffee enema stimulates the activity of this system by 600- 700%.

Coffee Enema Procedure

- This enema is retained for 12-14 minutes, during this time blood circulates in liver three times and blood is purified. Coffee enema can be given several times a day, few patients take up to seven times a day. Normally if pain is not relieved it may be taken more than one time. You should relax while taking enema; you may listen to music or read newspaper while relaxing. The best time for coffee enema is either early morning after you passed motion or during the day time.

- Grind organic coffee beans. Put approx. 750ml of filtered water in a steal pan and bring it to boil. Add 2-5 heaped Tbsp coffee powder, 3 Tbsp is ideal. It is roughly 20-25grams. Let it continue to simmer for ten minutes or more and then turn off the burner. Allow it to cool down to a very comfortable, tepid temperature. Test it with your finger. It should be the same temperature as your body's temperature. Filter the coffee with fine mesh steal sieve into a jug. This is approximately 500ml.

- Pour 2 cups (500ml) of coffee into the enema pot. Be sure the plastic hose is clamped tightly. Now open the clamp and grasp, but do not close the clamp on the hose. Place the enema tip in the sink. Hold up the enema bag above the tip until the coffee begins to flow out. As soon as it starts flowing, quickly close the clamp. This expels any air in the tube.

- Lubricate the enema tip with a small amount of coconut oil or KY jelly. Create a comfortable and relaxing atmosphere. After a few days you will thoroughly enjoy this ritual.

- Light a candle, play some light music and most importantly, make sure you are comfortable and warm.

We recommend placing a pillow with a washable cover under your head and lying down on an old towel.

- The position preferred is lying on your back. With the clamp closed hang the pot about 3 feet above your belly. We like to hang the enema pot on a drip stand.
- Insert the tip gently into anus and open the clamp slowly. You should relax and breathe. The coffee may take a few seconds to begin flowing. If you develop a cramp, close the hose clamp, turn from side to side and take a few deep breaths. The cramp will usually pass quickly. Usually nothing happens.
- When all the liquid is inside, close the clamp and remove it slowly. Retain the enema for 12- 14 minutes. You may remain lying on the floor.
- After 14 minutes or so, go to the toilet and empty your gut. Take your time. Wash the enema pot and tube thoroughly with soap and water.
- Take more potassium in the form of fruits and vegetable juices if you take coffee enema regularly (S.A.Wilsons.com).

Epsom bath

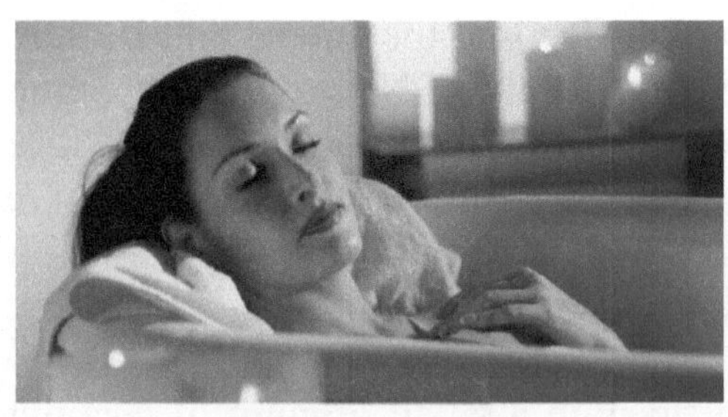

Detoxification of your body through bathing is an ancient remedy that anyone can perform in the comfort of your own home. Your skin is known as the third kidney, and toxins are excreted through sweating. An Epsom salt bath is thought to assist your body in eliminating toxins as well as absorbing the magnesium and nutrients that are in the water. Soaking in Epsom salt actually helps replenish the body's magnesium levels, combating hypertension. The sulfate flushes toxins and helps form proteins in brain tissue and joints. Most of all, it will leave you relaxed, refreshed and awakened. Take it once a week or as advised.

Prepare your bath

- It is a 40 minutes ritual. The first 20 minutes are said to help your body remove the toxins, while the second 20 minutes are for absorbing the minerals from the water
- Fill your tub with comfortably hot water. Use a chlorine filter if possible.
- Add Epsom salt (Magnesium sulfate). For people 50 Kg and up, add 2 cups or more to a standard bath tub.
- Then add 2 cups or more of soda bicarb. It is known for its cleansing ability and even has anti-fungal properties. It also leaves skin very soft.
- Add 2-3 Tbsp ground ginger. While this step is optional, ginger can increase your heat levels, helping to sweat out more toxins. However, since it is heating the body, it may cause your skin to turn slightly red for a few minutes, so be careful with the amount you add. Depending on the capacity of your tub, anywhere from 1 Tbsp to 1/3 cup can be added (Herneise).
- Add aromatherapy oils. Again optional, but there are many oils that will make the bath an even more pleasant and relaxing experience (such as lavender), as well as those that will assist in the detoxification process (tea tree or eucalyptus oil). Around 20 drops is sufficient for a standard bath.
- Swish all of the ingredients around in the tub, and then slip into the tub. You should start sweating within the first few minutes. If you feel too hot, start adding cold water into the tub until you cool off.
- Get out of the tub slowly and carefully. Your body has been working hard and you may get lightheaded or feel

weak and drained. On top of that, the salts make your tub slippery, so stand with care.

- Drink plenty of water and relax in bed for a few minutes

Soda bicarb bath

Lothar Hirneise has given lot of importance to Soda bicarb bath. It is thought to assist you in eliminating toxins as well as making your body alkaline so your tumor cells may suffocate. Patient may take it once or even twice a day. Just add 2 cups of soda bicarb in your bath tub filled with warm water and relax in it for 30-40 minutes (Hirneise, 2005).

Sun Therapy

Getting an adequate amount of sunshine is a critical part of Budwig protocol. Once the body has acquired the right oil-protein balance with the Cottage Cheeseand Flax oil, the body develops better capacity to absorb the healing photons from the sun. Remember that for healing of cancer high energy photons from the sun are very important. The sunshine is important to maintain adequate vitamin-D levels in our body. Vitamin-D is a powerful antioxidant that has been linked to preventing many diseases including cancer.

Dr. Budwig's focus was on the importance of photons from the sunbeams and their interaction with vital essential fats (linoleic and linolenic acid) in our body. It is the interaction of photons from the sun and the electrons in proper food that provide the synergistic effect on healing our body. Eating the electron rich Flax oil/Cottage Cheese mixture, must be connected with adequate exposure to sunlight.

There is nothing else on earth with a higher concentration of photons of the sun's energy than man. This concentration of the sun's energy is very much energetic point for humans, with their wave eminently suitable lengths - is improved when we eat electron rich essential oils, which in turn absorbs the photons in the form of electro-magnetic waves of sunbeams.

When you eat the FO/CC mixture, your body becomes a better antenna for the photons from the sunbeam. Your body develops a better ability to absorb the energy from the sun and Transfer it to your cells to perform their vital functions. You become energized at a deep level, and when this happens cancer is healed itself.

It is red light that penetrates deeper in the tissues. In 1968 Dr. Budwig used 695 nm ruby (red) lasers light with success to radiate healthy surrounding cancer tissues in cancer patients.

How long should you take this protocol?

If all is well patient feels better and tumor start to shrink within a 3 or 4 months, if he follows treatment religiously and honestly. He may be cured in one or two years. **It is recommended that the Budwig protocol and full diet is followed for at least five years.** Even after that he should maintain healthy eating and life style.

Dr. Budwig has clearly mentioned that if you do not get the desired success, do not blame the protocol, rather try to find out your mistakes and correct them. The threshold between winning and losing is very small, and even a minor mistake can unbalance the complete healing process.

Linomel

Linomel is an invention by Dr Budwig. Freshly crushed Flax seed is mixed with honey and milk powder so that the crushed Flax seed is more stable. There is no doubt that freshly crushed Flax seed is more valuable, but also has the disadvantage that you do it yourself and clean the grinder afterwards. That is why Linomel still has an existence right. Do not buy crushed Flax seed in the shop as the chance that these contain Trans fatty acids is 100%.

Is there an alternative to Linomel?
- Freshly crushed Flax seed is an alternative. This must be eaten immediately after the meal, otherwise it will oxidize.
- Make your own Linomel. Mix 6 tablespoons freshly crushed Flax seed with a tablespoon of honey. Small tip: Grind the Flax seed, e.g. in a coffee grinder, and set the grinder to coarse. So it mixes better with the honey.

(Oil Protein Diet by Lothar Hieneise)

Daylight

Dr Budwig focused upon the importance of daylight to our health. It is not enough to absorb electrons only through food, but it is important that we feed ourselves so that our cells are able to absorb and process the light coming from the sun. The more sickly someone is, the sooner he is "in the house", which can be a catastrophic mistake. Especially when people are already in a very late stage of the illness, they are often not able to eat enough and good advice is then very difficult. In such cases, Dr Budwig advises to concentrate on the following three points:

- ELDI oils as whole body rubbings and if possible as enemas
- Only freshly squeezed juices and distributed as food throughout the day if possible the breakfast muesli in different variants
- Stay outside as much as possible

You will experience me to explain what to do next. I have been able to see in my life how Dr Budwig's theoretical considerations work when put to practice, if indeed, if they are consistently carried out. If you could experience such a case yourself, and how quickly it can be better for a seriously ill person, you can see Dr Budwig's words in a very different light.

But other great researchers had also dealt with the subject of light long before Dr Budwig. For example, the anthroposophist Rudolf Steiner wrote, about 50 years earlier that there is a fundamental being of our material existence of the earth, of which all materiality has come only through condensation. Every matter on earth is condensed light! There is nothing in material existence, which is something else than condensed light in some form. Wherever you go and feel matter, you have condensed light everywhere. Compressed light. Matter is light by its very nature.

In as much as a man is a material being, he is woven of light. Rudolf Steiner and Dr Budwig have pointed out in their writings over and over again the importance of light and that we humans are now heliotropes, which need light and use light. But I have nowhere else than with Dr Budwig so clearly and understandably read, WHY this is and above all, how the charging of the life battery works and / or what importance mainly the linolenic acid or electron clouds play. Because it is so important, I would like to repeat here again: The sicklier someone is, the more he should be in the open." (Oil-Protein Diet by Lothar Hirneise)

Disclaimer

This book is not intended to replace the advice and/or care of a qualified health care professional. Please do not try to self diagnose or self treat any disease. Seek professional help and consult your physician before making any dietary changes.

This book is not intended to provide medical advice and is sold with the understanding that the publisher and the author have neither liability nor responsibility to any person or entity with respect to loss, damage or injury caused or alleged to be caused directly or indirectly by the information contained in this book or the use of any products mentioned. Readers should not use any of the product discussed in this book without the advice of a medical profession.

The Food and Drug Administration has not approved the use of any of the natural treatments discussed in this book. This book, and the information contained herein, has not been approved by the Food and the Drug Administration.

Cancer - Cause and Cure
Based on Quantum Physics developed by Dr. Johanna Budwig

http://www.amazon.com/Cancer-Quantum-Physics-developed-Johanna-ebook/dp/B00P3Y7BYG

Book Description

***** A must have book for every cancer patient *****

This book provides an introduction of Dr. Budwig's cancer research and treatment. Johanna

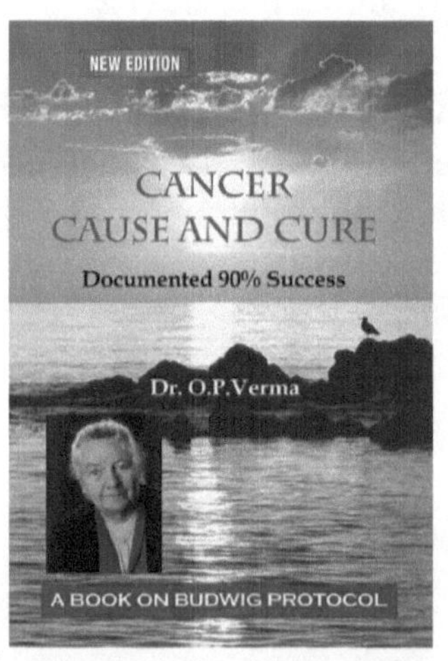

Budwig (1908-2003) was nominated for the Nobel Prize seven times. She was one of Germany's leading scientists of the 20th Century, a biochemist and cancer specialist with a special interest in essential fats.

Otto Warburg proved that prime cause of cancer oxygen-deficiency in the cells. In absence of oxygen cells ferment glucose to produce energy, lactic acid is formed as a byproduct of fermentation. He postulated that sulfur containing protein and some unknown fat is required to attract oxygen in the cell.

In 1951 Dr. Budwig developed Paper Chromatography to identify fats. With this technique she proved that electron rich highly unsaturated Linoleic and Linolenic fatty acids were the undiscovered mysterious decisive fats in respiratory enzyme function that Otto Warburg had been unable to find. She studied the electromagnetic function of pi-electrons of the linolenic acid in the membranes of the microstructure of protoplasm, for all nerve function, secretions, mitosis, as well as cell break-down. This immediately caused lot of excitement in the scientific community. New doors could open in Cancer research. Hydrogenated fats, including all Trans fatty acids were proved as respiratory poisons.

Then Budwig decided to have human trials and gave flaxseed oil and quark to cancer patients. After three months, the patients began to improve in health and strength, the yellow green substance in their blood began to disappear, tumors gradually receded and at the same time the nutrients began to rise. This way Dr. Budwig had found a cure for cancer. It was a great victory and first milestone in the battle against cancer. Her treatment protocol is based on the consumption of flax seed oil with low fat cottage cheese, raw organic diet, mild exercise, and the healing powers of the sun. She treated approx. 2500 cancer patients during a 50 year period with this protocol till her death with over 90% documented success.

She was nominated 7 times for Nobel Prize but with a condition that she will use chemotherapy and radiotherapy with her protocol. They did not want to collapse the 200 billion dollar business over night. She always refused to support the damaging chemo and radio for the sake of humanity.

The book also, describes about rare and miraculous herbs used in the treatment of Cancer like Turmeric, Black seed, Ginger, Mistle Toe, Aloe vera, Echinecea, Lobelia, Essiac Tea, Pau d'arco Tea, Dandelion, Milk Thistle.

~~**~~

Cancer Cure Is Found: Letrile is the answer

https://www.amazon.com/Cancer-Cure-Found-Laetrile-answer/dp/1797710206/

CANCER CURE IS FOUND

During 1950, a biochemist Dr. Ernest T. Krebs Jr., isolated a new vitamin from bitter apricot kernel that he called 'B-17' or 'Laetrile'. He conducted further lab animal and culture experiments to conclude that laetrile would be effective in the treatment of cancer. He proposed that cancer was caused by a deficiency of Vitamin B 17 (Laetrile, Amygdaline). Laetrile is a concentrated and purified form of vitamin B17. After a lot of research, he had finally developed a specific protocol to treat cancer. Laetrile Therapy combines Laetrile with nutritional supplements and a healthy diet to create a potent treatment that fights cancer cells while helping to strengthen the body's immune system.

Vitamin B-17, which is present in several different foods, consists of a locked substance which comprises two units' glucose, one unit benzaldehyde and one unit cyanide. When B17 comes in contact with a cancer cell it is unlocked by a hormone found only in the cancer cell, and becomes a lethal chemical bomb which destroys the cancer cell. Healthy cells do not cause breakdown of B17. Cancer is unknown to people living in areas with food products rich in B-17, and the population lives to a remarkably high age. Apparently nature has provided us with an ingenious defense against cancer, and it is an ordinary nutrient in

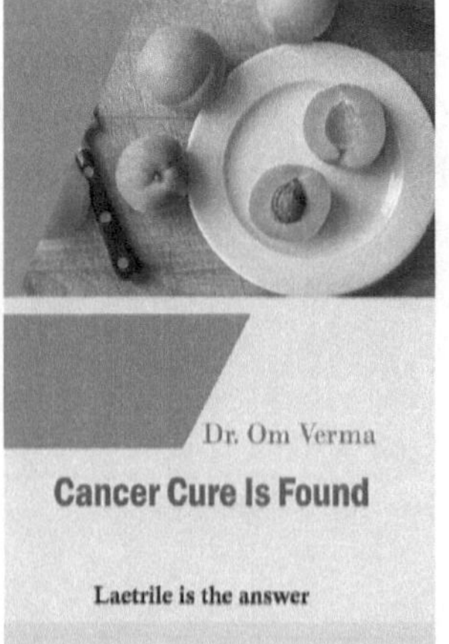

our food. These are, amongst others nuts, seeds, vegetables, and in particular apricot kernels.

At present, patients listen or read a lot about Laetrile treatment, but usually they don't get precise and to the point information about what are the exact components of this protocol, where to get Laetrile injections and supplements, what to take, what not to take, what are the doses, how long to take the treatment, what diet they have to follow, etc. In this book, I have explained the protocol in detail proposed by Dr. Krebs. I have given every minute detail about Laetrile, other nutritional supplements and diet in this book. After reading this book patients can buy Laetrile injections, tablets and other nutritional supplements from the reliable sources (given in the book) and conduct the treatment under the supervision of their family doctor. Dr. Philip E. Binzel was personally trained by Dr. Ernest T. Kreb Jr. about everything of this treatment. Dr. Binzel had been using Laetrile therapy in the treatment of cancer patients since the mid 1970s. His record of success was astounding. Testimonies of his patients are also included in this book.